Praise for *Field E*

Anyone with the desire to truly understa...
stress of being in service has had on veterans but the incredible transfor-
mational impact being in nature has on healing them should read this
book. In truth though, everyone can benefit from reading *Field Exercises*, as it is rich with wisdom and information that can reconnect all of
us back to our nature as beings who are deeply connected to the earth.

—Eva Selhub, MD Specialist in Mind-Body Medicine, Inspiration Teacher and
Resiliency Coach. Author, *The Love Response* and *Your Brain on Nature.*
Instructor in Medicine Harvard Medical School,
Clinical Associate Massachusetts General Hospital

Field Exercises is an not only an outstanding synthesis of state of the art
research concerning natural environments and human-animal bonds - it
is brought to life by its reflection off the emotionally raw, deeply moving accounts of veterans. The result of this combination, guided by the
beautiful writing style of Dr. Westlund and the poignant, intelligent,
experience-based words of veterans, is a call to action. If we want to
Support our Troops, we should listen to them. *Field Exercises* makes it
clear that they have much to teach all of us concerning social capital, resilience, sustainability, biodiversity, physical activity, mindfulness, and
how these and other factors intersect with ecosystem services and the
global metal health crisis.

—Alan C. Logan, co-author, *Your Brain on Nature*

If we are right, the current wave of veterans coming home from war and
entering into Agriculture will only continue to grow. When it does, then
Field Exercises will have been one of the first looks at the complicated
mix of motivations that have called veterans to serve their country again
as farmers.

—Michael O'Gorman, Founder and Director, Farmer Veteran Coalition

The almost constant combat since 9/11 has taken a substantial toll on many of the men and women who have served their nation with selfless dedication. In her book, *Field Exercises*, Stephanie Westlund has done a wonderful job of capturing the intensely personal battles some veterans continue to fight upon their return home, while simultaneously shining a light on the transformative power that nature can have for those willing to embrace it. Her thoroughly-researched book builds a powerful case for continuing to explore alternative nature-based activities as part of a broader effort to support veterans as they search to find peace at home as a result of conflict in far-off lands.

—Chad Spangler, National Director, Outward Bound Veterans

field
EXERCISES

How Veterans Are
Healing Themselves through
Farming and Outdoor Activities

Stephanie Westlund

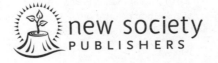

new society
PUBLISHERS

Cover design by Diane McIntosh. Cover photos: top left: CVAF Rafting Trip, 2009, Inside Out Experience (insideoutexperience.com); top right: Harvesting Carrots at Growing Veterans, 2013, Nick Gonzales (NickGphotos.com); center and back cover: Trail Ride, 2010, Christian McEachern; bottom: Picking Tomatoes at Growing Veterans, 2013, Nick Gonzales (NickGphotos.com)

Printed in Canada. First printing June 2014.

This book is intended for informational purposes only, and does not constitute a substitute for medical or psychiatric advice. Neither the publisher nor the author accepts any responsibility for the outcomes of any activities carried out by anyone else as a result, direct or indirect, of reading this book.

New Society Publishers acknowledges the financial support of the Government of Canada through the Canada Book Fund (CBF) for our publishing activities.

Inquiries regarding requests to reprint all or part of *Field Exercises* should be addressed to New Society Publishers at the address below.

To order directly from the publishers, please call toll-free (North America) 1-800-567-6772, or order online at www.newsociety.com

Any other inquiries can be directed by mail to:

New Society Publishers
P.O. Box 189, Gabriola Island, BC V0R 1X0, Canada
(250) 247-9737

LIBRARY AND ARCHIVES CANADA CATALOGUING IN PUBLICATION

Westlund, Stephanie, author
Field exercises : how veterans are healing themselves through farming and outdoor activities / Stephanie Westlund.

Includes bibliographical references and index.
Issued in print and electronic formats.
ISBN 978-0-86571-761-9 (pbk.).—ISBN 978-1-55092-556-2 (ebook)

1. Post-traumatic stress disorder—Alternative treatment.
2. Veterans—Mental health.   3. Nature, Healing power of.
4. Agriculture—Therapeutic use.   5. Gardening—Therapeutic use.
6. Outdoor recreation—Therapeutic use.   I. Title.

RC451.4.V48W38 2014   616.85'212   C2014-902315-4
C2014-902316-2

New Society Publishers' mission is to publish books that contribute in fundamental ways to building an ecologically sustainable and just society, and to do so with the least possible impact on the environment, in a manner that models this vision. We are committed to doing this not just through education, but through action. The interior pages of our bound books are printed on Forest Stewardship Council®-registered acid-free paper that is 100% post-consumer recycled (100% old growth forest-free), processed chlorine-free, and printed with vegetable-based, low-VOC inks, with covers produced using FSC®-registered stock. New Society also works to reduce its carbon footprint, and purchases carbon offsets based on an annual audit to ensure a carbon neutral footprint. For further information, or to browse our full list of books and purchase securely, visit our website at: www.newsociety.com

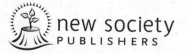

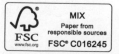

For all who suffer,
and for the fallen and their families.

⊕ ⊕ ⊕

CONTENTS

ACKNOWLEDGMENTS

A book such as this requires time and effort from so many people, and it's impossible to express the extent of my gratitude to all who have been involved. First and foremost, thank you to those whose stories are contained herein: Christian McEachern, Deston Denniston, Penny Dex, Shepherd Bliss, Nathan Lewis, Christopher Brown, Gordon Cousins, Steve Critchley and Jim Marland. I am humbled by your trust in me, and you have my utmost respect for the work you do every day. On days when writing this book seemed to be an impossible task, I drew inspiration from you and from knowing that your stories matter to the world. You have taught me so much. To all the others who graciously gave their time to be interviewed, thank you. And my appreciation to Michael Parmeley for granting permission to include his poem.

Deston Denniston gets all the credit for the main *Field Exercises* title—and thank you to all others who gave their thoughts and advice. Thank you, too, to Inside Out Experience, Christian McEachern, Nick Gonzales and Growing Veterans for the cover photos, and to the photographers who generously donated the photos for the book chapters.

To the New Society team, thank you for your enthusiasm and for working with me to make this book a reality—especially Ingrid Witvoet, Sue Custance and EJ Hurst for responding tirelessly to all my questions through the process. And my full gratitude to my editor Betsy Nuse for her thoughtful and sensitive edits and advice.

To my early readers Audrey Smith, Jackie Seidel and Scott Westlund, I truly appreciated your time, honesty and suggestions. And to Deston, Christian, Penny, Shepherd, Nathan, Gordon, Christopher, Steve and Jim, for taking the time to carefully review your own chapters, thank you.

Although now greatly different in both content and form, some of the initial research for this book came out of my doctoral studies in Peace and Conflict Studies at the University of Manitoba's Arthur V. Mauro Centre for Peace and Justice. Particular thanks go to Jessica Senehi, Marlene Atleo, Shirley Thompson and Sean Byrne for supporting that work. I also recognize the Social Sciences and Humanities Research Council of Canada for their financial support during my doctoral studies. And my gratitude to the University of Calgary's Consortium for Peace Studies, which granted me the 2012–2013 Arthur Clark Research Fellowship in Global Citizenship so that I could continue to do research and interviews for this book.

Thanks and love to the many family members and friends who have supported this journey. Special thanks to my parents Fritz and Hanne, my in-laws Kirk and Sharon and my sister Katie for helping with child care, and to the many other wonderful caregivers who have allowed me time to focus on my research and writing.

My deepest gratitude goes to my partner Scott and son Cameron, who spent many weekends out of the house so that I could write. Scott, I couldn't have done it without your love, support and constant encouragement. And Cameron, who has spent more time in the university library than most toddlers, thank you for your unconditional love and joyful presence and for providing lots of playtime to keep me grounded in the world!

Introduction

We are human only in contact,
and conviviality, with what is not human.
DAVID ABRAM

"In the military, we're taught to be given a task, to see to that task, and to complete that task. And it's been hard with prolonged warfare for service members to see the completion of a task, to see something through. I think there are very negative psychological consequences to that," said Tia Christopher, a US Navy veteran and now Chief of Staff for the Farmer Veteran Coalition. "We've found that when veterans can follow a plant cycle—when they prepare the earth, they plant the seed, they nurture it, they harvest it, and they eat it or they sell it—that process in itself is healing." Farming, Tia explained, can offer "alternative therapy that isn't therapy. I always say that the sweat of their backs and working in the soil and working with the animals really helps veterans heal."[1]

Tia Christopher's comments may explain the growing momentum amongst veterans throughout North America who are finding relief from stressful and traumatic military experiences through outdoor activities, from farming and gardening to hiking, canoeing and spending time with horses and dogs. *Field Exercises* tells the compelling stories of veterans from different generations who have discovered that their suffering is eased by contact with nature.[2] Their stories illuminate the courage required to live with and recover from experiences of violence and trauma, while also offering hope and possibility for others seeking additional methods to ease the transition to civilian life, manage injuries and recover from military stress and trauma.

Nature-based health care approaches are largely unacknowledged in North America, despite a growing body of empirical research that supports them and the fact that many people are individually realizing the importance of nature contact in their lives. *Field Exercises* is a call for wider support for programs that bring farming, gardening and other outdoor activities to soldiers and veterans. "It's not the silver bullet but almost across the board, in every case, nature contact matters," said Keith Tidball, a former US National Guard infantry officer-turned-academic, who studies veterans and outdoor recreation. For veterans and active duty soldiers, "any kind of nature exposure will be helpful."[3]

Connecting with nature, however, does not in itself guarantee transformation or healing and recovery, and nature contact is not a cure-all or magic treatment for veterans.[4] Indeed, I recently learned about a veteran whose post-traumatic stress symptoms are triggered by the smell of dirt, which would make farming, gardening and many other outdoor activities difficult for him. Many veterans are also finding other activities and therapies to be important in their lives, ranging from medication and psychotherapy to writing and volunteering. Based on his own psychotherapy practice, Edward Tick observed that post-traumatic stress is best recognized as "an identity disorder and soul wound." And understood this way, Tick has suggested that the symptoms of the injury diminish when veterans connect to the sacredness of life, through purification rituals, storytelling, healing journeys, amongst other rituals and ceremonies.[5] *Field Exercises* reveals how farming and outdoor activities might also provide a sacred connection to life for many veterans.

Why I Wrote This Book

Veterans often wonder why a civilian would want to write this book. The seeds were first planted in 2004, when I watched the documentary *Shake Hands with the Devil: The Journey of Roméo Dallaire*, a devastating account of the United Nations Assistance Mission for Rwanda's failure to prevent the Rwandan genocide.[6] In the years since, Canadian Lieutenant General (retired) Roméo Dallaire, who was commander of the mission, has spoken openly and candidly about his post-traumatic struggles. In the film, Dallaire returned to Rwanda for the 10-year commemoration of the genocide, and there is a scene halfway through when Dallaire and his wife Élizabeth stand holding hands atop a lush terraced hillside, a place he visited often during the mission. He tells her, "C'est ici que j'ai redevenu humain" (English translation: "It's here that I became human again"). Later, Dallaire returned with the filmmakers to that hilltop and remarked, "I want to show you where in all this I could find myself. I could find the solace and be one with my soul, with my heart, with my being." At the time, these two scenes provoked me to reflect upon the serenity and calm beauty of that hillside contrasted with the extreme violence that occurred in and around it in 1994. But it wasn't until several years later, while working on my doctoral research in Peace and Conflict Studies, that I became conscious of how often the images of LGen Dallaire standing on that hillside returned to mind.

A second seed came while reading neurologist and psychiatrist Viktor Frankl's account of his experiences in Nazi death camps during World War II; it provides several glimpses into how hope and solace are found in human beings' relationships with nature, even under desperate circumstances.[7] Frankl described how even in a concentration camp, prisoners would draw one another's attention to the beauty of a sunset. And he recalled another time, when he and a group of prisoners were being transferred by train from Auschwitz to a camp in Bavaria, "If someone had seen our faces on the journey...as we beheld the mountains of Salzburg with their summits glowing in the sunset, through the little barred windows of the prison carriage," Frankl wrote, "he would never have believed that those were the faces of men who had given up all hope of life and liberty. Despite that factor—or maybe because of it—we were carried away by nature's beauty, which we had missed for so long."[8]

I have since come across many similar stories. For example, Canadian scholar Harold Adams Innis was wounded as a young soldier during World War I. In 1924, Innis undertook a summer-long canoe trip on the Peace and Slave Rivers with his friend John Long. Innis's biographer, Donald Creighton, wrote that "the long summer, with its wind and sun, its space, and peace, and friendly companionship, had done [Innis] an immense amount of good. He had, as it were, shaken off the last of the evil effects of the war.... He had recovered his health and spirits."[9]

Throughout history, gardens have been cultivated around the world under the most extreme circumstances and in the most unexpected places. Kenneth Helphand's book *Defiant Gardens* offers a glimpse of gardens planted and nurtured during wartime by soldiers, ghetto residents, prisoners of war and internees in the first half of the 20th century.[10] Soldiers in World War I even planted and harvested gardens right in the trenches, which Helphand argued demonstrated their "struggle to create something normal in the most abnormal conditions."[11] Such gardens also represented soldiers' hope that a future was possible.

During the early 20th century, *garden therapy* was incorporated into the treatment regime for US soldiers suffering from shell-shock.[12] At the end of World War I, the US military implemented a number of gardening treatment programs for veterans.[13] Influential US psychiatrist Karl Menninger, who along with his father F.C. Menninger founded the Menninger Foundation in Topeka, Kansas, strongly advocated for horticulture therapy to support veterans in recovering from their experiences in World War II.[14] In fact, the horticulture therapy movement, which today works with a wide clientele, first became organized in the US around work in veterans' hospitals.[15] Menninger viewed horticulture therapy as holding possibilities for bringing "the individual close to the soil and close to Mother Nature, close to beauty, close to the inscrutable mystery of growth and development."[16]

In 1942, the Canadian government instituted the *Veterans' Land Act*, which provided grants and low-interest loans for veterans to become farmers, smallholders and commercial fishermen. The loans and grants were provided for purchasing land, farm equipment and livestock. Veterans were also given access to agricultural training, both through hands-on training with other farmers and in the form of information and lessons from instructors and inspectors. The program supported more than 140,000 Canadian veterans before being terminated in 1977.[17]

As part of my doctoral research in Peace and Conflict Studies, I interviewed veterans who are finding that nature supports them in managing their post-traumatic stress symptoms. All described how contact with nature gave them the space to voice their suffering, to develop resiliency, to have meaningful conversations about their experiences and to find ways to continue living their lives. All spoke about their continued desire to serve their communities, and through their individual work, began creating a social foundation to support others in also moving toward healing. Deeply moved by the veterans' courage and personal resolve to move through pain toward recovery, I vowed to bring these stories to a wider audience.

Interviewing veterans has been a reminder of the fragility of all life. War and other forms of political violence directly affect all people on the planet—soldiers and civilians alike. Lives, relationships and families are harmed and destroyed by extended cycles of violence and conflict. Yet as I have worked on *Field Exercises*, I have come to realize the deep disconnect between the North American civilian understanding of war and the experiences of military service members. Most civilians have little awareness of the activities and experiences of military personnel. Moreover, unless they have direct contact with someone who suffers from post-traumatic stress, they have little sympathy for the invisible wounds of war; they have difficulty understanding why recovery isn't a more immediate process. Civilians tend to uphold many stereotypes about veterans, including a sense that veterans can be a risk to their communities—a perception often sensationalized and exacerbated by the media but which is generally untrue. As Greg Prodaniuk, the western regional coordinator for the Operational Stress Injury support program in Canada, has explained, "The vast majority of them suffer in silence and in their basements, and they don't hurt people.... But they do destroy relationships.... They have difficulty controlling their emotions. They have reactions they're not in control of."[18]

The third reason I wrote this book is because of my own experiences with and in nature. I spent most of my childhood in rural Alberta, much of that time outdoors, trekking in and around swamps, lakes, rivers, forests and brush, stacking wood for fires, canoeing, camping, cross-country skiing, riding horses and pursuing small critters. These experiences gave me a deep understanding that human life was connected with the natural world. In my occasional university teaching, I have also experimented with taking students outside. In this age of laptop computers, tablets and cell phones, most students are continuously plugged in and distracted by their electronic devices inside the classroom; when we go outside together, sit in small groups on the grass, surrounded by pine and deciduous trees, feeling the sun and a light breeze on our skin, students put these devices away without being asked and genuinely focus on one another. Compared with the days we stay in our windowless classroom, when we go outside together, students seem to engage in better discussions and develop deeper and more intimate connections with one another. For the past four years, I have also seen how, for my young son, nature is enchanting at every possible turn, in stories, toys and outdoor play. And I often wonder, at what point do animals and rocks and trees, pinecones and leaves, the moon and stars lose their voices and only become the passive backdrop to our human lives?

For the veterans in this book, nature is not a passive backdrop. It has become an active participant in their lives. And both veterans and non-veterans can learn much from these stories of reestablishing relationships with the wider world—about what is fundamentally important to us as human beings and our psyches, and the ways we are not separate from the world of nature. The veterans provide deep insight into the human-nature relationship, and through them, other military personnel and their families, and civilians, too, might find additional ways to cope with and manage their injuries, reduce their suffering and support soldiers' transition to civilian life.

Accordingly, this book is an offering, intended to gather support and bring awareness, in military and civilian communities alike, about the importance of nature contact. It tells of the relief that veterans are personally finding and investigates how their anecdotal reports have support from a growing body of empirical research. Veterans are doing this work in spite of the regular and significant challenges they encounter from day to day—and this work often helps some of the personal difficulties fade, even if only momentarily. They passionately persevere in their endeavors regardless of the obstacles, and as I argue in the final chapter of *Field Exercises*, they are at the forefront of a veteran-led movement for green care in North America. But despite their passion, success is not assured, and veterans need wider community support.

The veterans who participated were chosen for the ways their stories provide insight into different aspects of military and post-military experience. Each chapter is based on multiple recorded interviews and is written in the veteran's voice as much as possible, with a focus primarily on recovery efforts. Each veteran was invited to read drafts of his/her chapter and to help decide which parts of his/her experience would be included in the book. It is important to remember that these stories reflect a certain time in the life of each person, and those lives continue to change and move forward day by day, year by year. By the time you are reading their stories, some details and aspects will have changed.

Meditation on
Being a Baby Killer

We knew that we killed them
although no one had said it,
the terrified mother
clutching terrified child.

Big Sherman, my gunner,
said he couldn't continue.
He'd looked in the bunker.
He started to cry.

I tell him, "It happens.
No one had meant it.
It happens in war.
We have to move on."

Time passes, much later;
the bunker's behind me.
In my mind I revisit.
I try to move on.

Somewhere inside me
Big Sherman is crying.
I tell him it happens.
I tell myself too.

There's a myth of recovery,
that you put it behind you,
remember the good times,
let bad memories fade.

But memories aren't like that.
Like bones they help build you.
They stand up to be counted.
They're part of what's true.

And now I'm a writer.
I put words on paper,
like baby and bunker
and terrified mother.

I know that we killed them.
No one need say it.
I know that they're dying
right now as I speak.

A mother and child,
alone in a bunker,
a war passing over,
right now as I speak.

Michael Parmeley,
Vietnam combat veteran[1]

1

Transitioning to Civilian Life and Living with Post-Traumatic Stress

There are many reasons men and women enlist in the military: it might be a calling, family tradition, economic opportunities lacking at home or patriotism. Some just want to experience the seeming adventure of military lifestyle; some fall into it because recruiters tell them being a soldier is just like camping (the infantry at least); for some enlisting seems like a natural progression from Cadets. Most soldiers also attest to a strong desire to serve their communities. But few who enlist in the military imagine they might experience deep, lasting and invisible wounds from war. While the risks of physical injury, and even death, are ever present and perhaps weigh on their minds, trauma exposure, stress reactions and post-traumatic stress are generally not at the forefront of consideration; service members might be aware of the possibility, but never imagine it will happen to them. However, for many military personnel (some estimates are as high as 25 to 30%), invisible injuries become a profound reality.

All who serve in the military are changed by the experience, and the transition to civilian (and veteran) is often a profound time in a soldier's life accompanied by intense and overwhelming confusion, instability and restlessness. The veteran needs not only to make sense of his or her experiences in the military, but also to develop a new identity outside the military and find a place in civilian society.[2] Despite these challenges, however, there is a societal expectation for soldiers to make the transition quickly and easily.

These challenges are compounded for veterans who are also wounded—physically, psychologically and/or spiritually and morally. And while many veterans do make a successful transition, others struggle for various reasons and to varying degrees. Many find that their skills and training do not easily transfer; they have difficulty finding work in the civilian sector. In the US, it's estimated that there are currently more than 200,000 unemployed Iraq and Afghanistan veterans.[3] Some military personnel experience a significant decline in income during the transition period. A Canadian study, for example, revealed that most Regular Forces veterans experienced a 10% drop in income after leaving the military, but this percentage was significantly higher for certain populations: female veterans experienced on average a 30% decline in income and medically released personnel a 29% decline.[4]

Many also struggle with homelessness, or are at risk of becoming homeless. Canada does not track veteran homelessness,[5] but in both the US and the UK, 25% of the homeless population are veterans; in the US, this amounts to nearly 200,000 homeless veterans![6] Further, the National Coalition for Homeless Veterans estimates that as many as 1.5 million US veterans are "at risk of homelessness due to poverty, lack of support networks and dismal, overcrowded, living conditions."[7]

Published nearly 40 years after he led a combat platoon in Vietnam, Michael Parmeley's poem, which begins this chapter, invites us into his experience as a twenty-one-year-old infantry lieutenant. Parmeley captured the unexpectedness of unimaginable trauma, and shared his 40-year-long struggle with emotions and memories of his involvement in the deaths of a mother and child. He also exposed the misnomer of recovery and powerfully challenged the notions that veterans should "just get over it," "suck it up," "move on" or simply forget about their wartime experiences.

In his book *Warrior Rising*, LCol Chris Linford wrote, "The military is very good at teaching us how to fight and survive in war zones but they have not taught us to survive what we saw and did in those war zones."[8] As Shepherd Bliss, one of the veterans interviewed for this book, told me, "I think that's something people don't understand about moral injury:[9] you get rewired, and you can't just wish it away. You can work on it, but sometimes people think, why are you still grieving? Why are you still experiencing this? You can't just turn it off. It's gone into your brain cells and your body, and you can't totally go away from it."[10]

All the veterans who shared their stories for this book have had their lives forever changed by their military service, whether or not they participated in combat. Most were injured during their time in the military; some suffered physical injuries, and most also suffered invisible injuries. Some have experienced the unspeakable—and like Michael Parmeley—they can never escape these experiences, stresses and traumas. All are now working to find ways of living with how the military trained them and with what they witnessed, did and/or experienced. As Parmeley wrote, the events and traumas provide the context—the bones—of a veteran's present life: "They stand up to be counted. They're part of what's true."

The common adage that "time heals all wounds" often does not hold true for those living with stress injuries. Many veterans continue to suffer long-term, and for some, the symptoms become worse over time.[11] In 1992, 50 years after the Canadian Forces' assault at the beaches of Dieppe, it was estimated that 30–43% of the surviving veterans continued to suffer from post-traumatic stress.[12] And LGen (Ret'd) Roméo Dallaire has commented that part of the viciousness of post-traumatic stress is that the sufferer never knows when s/he will be reminded of and led down the path of revisiting previous trauma experiences;[13] stress injury symptoms can be triggered anywhere, anytime, by anything, ranging from sights to smells to sounds. There is no "off switch."

While LCol Chris Linford considers himself a post-traumatic stress disorder (PTSD) survivor, he wrote, "I still have to manage it from day to day."[14] And many World War II veterans experience as much distress today as they did nearly 70 years ago: they still don't sleep, they still have flashbacks and nightmares, they still weep over their experiences, and many recall the war as though it happened this morning.[15] Accordingly, while in this book I do use the terms recovery and healing, it is with an understanding that veterans' experiences will always be part of who they are, and that it's from and with these experiences that they move forward with their lives. The recovery of health can take many forms depending on the severity of veterans' injuries, but for the most part recovery does not mean cure.

From Disorder to Injury—A Brief History of Terminology

The English word "trauma" is the same as its Greek word of origin, *trauma*, meaning "wound," and in Western society, there has long been an understanding of the trauma inflicted by violent conflict. For thousands of years, symptoms of acute stress have been associated with and understood as part of soldiers' war experience. Psychiatrist Jonathan Shay described the ways that Homer's *Iliad* (800 BCE), which chronicles Achilles' experiences during the Trojan War, is an excellent account of the stress and trauma experienced by combat soldiers. Shay's work with Vietnam veterans revealed that many post-traumatic stress sufferers report living through most or all of the experiences documented in the *Iliad*: "a leader's betrayal of 'what's right,' blunted responsiveness to any emotional, social, or ethical claims outside a tiny circle of combat-proven comrades, grief and guilt for death(s) in this circle, lust for revenge, renunciation of ever returning home, seeing one's self as already dead, berserking, dishonoring the enemy, and loss of humanity."[16]

Other traumas of war were chronicled by Greek historian Herodotus (484–425 BCE), who described how the Athenian warrior Epizêlus was blinded during the Battle of Marathon "without blow of sword or dart" when the soldier next to him was killed.

> A strange prodigy likewise happened at this fight. Epizêlus, the son of Cuphagoras, an Athenian, was in the thick of the fray, and behaving himself as a brave man should, when suddenly he was stricken with blindness, without blow of sword or dart; and this blindness continued thenceforth during the whole of his after life. The following is the account which he himself, as I have heard, gave of the matter: he said that a gigantic warrior, with a huge beard, which shaded all his shield, stood over against him, but the ghostly semblance passed him by, and slew the man at his side. Such, as I understand, was the tale which Epizêlus told.[17]

The invisible wounds and anxiety that can arise from combat stress have been described using various terminologies. In the 17th century, Spanish doctors used the expression *estar roto*, literally meaning "to be broken."[18] During the US Civil War, it was called "soldier's heart."[19] The term "shell shock" first appeared in *The Lancet* in early 1915, a few months after the start of World War I.[20] Shell shock was initially considered to be a physical injury, resulting from a soldier's brain being shaken in his skull during a shell explosion. However, over the course of the war, psychiatrists began to see shell shock in increasing numbers of soldiers who had been nowhere near an explosion. When it was realized that these soldiers were suffering from emotional shock rather than physical trauma, they were often singled out as "cowards and traitors" by their peers and superiors, a stigma that many veterans suffering from post-traumatic stress continue to experience today.[21]

"Combat fatigue" and "battle fatigue" were the common terms used during World War II.[22] As evidenced by the word "fatigue," it was becoming better understood that war brought psychological trauma for many soldiers and other service personnel. According to the US government, approximately 10% (101 per 1000) of US soldiers in World War II suffered from combat-related fatigue.[23] However, the Director of the Harvard Program in Refugee Trauma, Richard F. Mollica, and his colleagues have suggested that twice as many soldiers suffered psychological wounds as physical wounds in World War I, and that in World War II, 33% of all wounds were of the invisible kind.[24]

The Vietnam War brought the term "post-Vietnam syndrome" into common usage.[25] In the 1960s and 1970s as psychiatrists worked with Vietnam veterans, they became increasingly sensitive to and sought to better understand how wartime experiences continued to affect the soldiers once they'd returned home. More than 80% of the time, as suggested by its name, post-Vietnam syndrome became part of the veteran's experience only once he had been discharged from the military and was trying to reintegrate into civilian life. While some Vietnam veterans were able to reintegrate into American society with relative ease, it was estimated that between 400,000 and 700,000 combat veterans encountered tremendous difficulties.[26] Some studies suggest that as many as 50% of Vietnam veterans suffered from some form of distress.[27]

Throughout the late 1960s and 1970s, as psychiatrists Chaim Sha-tan and Robert Jay Lifton worked with Vietnam veterans, they lobbied for a new diagnostic concept to be added to the American Psychiatric Association's official diagnostic manual.[28] It was during this time that post-traumatic stress disorder (PTSD) first became identified as a syndrome undeniably related to combat exposure, and in 1980 PTSD was officially added as a category to the *Diagnostic and Statistical Manual of Mental Disorders* (then the DSM-III).[29]

Since its addition to the DSM-III, PTSD has become recognized as a condition that affects not only combat soldiers and veterans. In Canada, recent reports show that a growing number of emergency professionals, such as firefighters and RCMP officers, are receiving a medical diagnosis of PTSD.[30] It also affects many people subjected to other forms of violence and trauma, including sexual and domestic violence, political violence and terror, and those who have lived through a natural disaster.[31] And complex humanitarian emergencies, in which many people are exposed to life-threatening events, can bring an increase in psychological suffering and PTSD.[32] Even witnesses to a violent act or accident, such as a motor vehicle accident, an airline disaster or a nuclear accident, as well as those who learn that something terrible has befallen a close relative or friend, may develop symptoms associated with PTSD.[33]

Importantly, not everyone who survives these situations will suffer from persistent PTSD, although symptoms can take months or years to emerge.[34] In general, the greatest risk for suffering seems to be exposure to interpersonal violence, particularly combat exposure and rape for men, and rape and being threatened with a weapon for women.[35] In addition, the more traumatic events to which a person is exposed, the greater the likelihood that they will experience and suffer distress.[36]

Within the academic and psychological/psychiatric communities, as well as amongst veterans themselves, there is now growing debate over the term "disorder." Many veterans object to it, since they consider their experiences of stress and distress to be an appropriate adaptation and response to the trauma and violence they have experienced and in which they have participated.

While the language around PTSD continues to be popular, the umbrella term "operational stress injury" (OSI) is now used within the Canadian Forces to describe "any persistent psychological difficulty resulting from operational duties performed while serving."[37] All peer-support clinics established by Veterans Affairs Canada are named Operational Stress Injury Clinics, and many veterans favor the expression operational stress injury because it "is less intimidating and emphasizes that the problem is an 'injury', not a mental disease."[38]

Jungian psychologist James Hillman, in his book *A Terrible Love of War*, contended that the stress of war should be considered inhuman, and argued that "the very idea that human agony can be named a 'stress syndrome' is inhuman, imagining a man as a machine part, a cog in a military wheel."[39] In searching for terminology outside the medical model, Hillman suggested becoming aware of how other expressions such as *estar roto* (to be broken), soldier's heart and shell shock all convey powerful images of shock and distress when compared with PTSD, which simply becomes an abbreviation or organizing category on a medical report.

In his keynote address as part of a Farmer Veteran Coalition event, Shepherd Bliss spoke to attendees about "farming as healing, especially for post-traumatic stress." He continued, "You'll notice I don't say post-traumatic stress disorder. It's not a disorder. It's an appropriate response to trauma."[40] During one of our conversations, Shepherd Bliss explained further:

> I don't like the term "PTSD" because the problem is then you see yourself as a disorder. Nobody is a disorder. I don't like the term "illegal immigrants." Nobody's illegal. So language is key. There is a shock there, and I think [shell shock] is a better term. And there is stress. But you don't have to image yourself as a victim. It's how not to be a victim, how to know that you hurt, admit you were hurt and not perpetuate it on the next generation or people—but somehow pick up your bed and walk, basically.[41]

Barbara Van Dahlen, founder of Give an Hour, a group of mental-health counselors working with veterans, is similarly adamant about abandoning the term "disorder": "They're going through a reasonable reaction to the terrifying experience of combat," she said recently.[42] And in a 2010 interview on PBS, psychiatrist Jonathan Shay suggested either "psychological injury" or "moral injury" as substitute terms. In particular, Shay said, moral injury happens when "there's the added dimension of betrayal of what's right by someone who holds legitimate authority in a high stakes situation." He argued that misconduct by a leader in a combat situation is often much more harmful than being shot at by an enemy.[43] Psychotherapist and ecopsychologist Andy Fisher has suggested the term "post-traumatic distress."[44]

I share these aversions to the term 'disorder," which blames the sufferer for traumatic experiences beyond their control. However, because PTSD continues to be commonly used, including by many veterans, it was difficult not to use it in this book. Accordingly, I follow each veteran's lead and use the term s/he uses. Elsewhere, I use the term "post-traumatic stress" (without disorder), although I use PTSD when referring to the medical literature.

Symptoms Commonly Associated with Post-Traumatic Stress

A person is medically diagnosed with PTSD only after their symptoms and distress have endured for more than one month.[45] As defined in both the American Psychiatric Association's *Diagnostic and Statistical Manual of Mental Disorders* (currently the DSM-5) and the World Health Organization's International Classification of Diseases (currently the ICD-10), the symptoms associated with PTSD include disturbing memories, nightmares, thought intrusions and physical sensations and flashbacks. Symptoms may come and go, and can be triggered by various life events. Triggers vary depending on the sensations the person experienced during the traumatic event(s). For example, many veterans are triggered by the smell of meat cooking on a barbeque, gas or diesel exhaust, garbage burning or blood. Others are triggered by loud noises, fireworks, helicopters or power tools. During a flashback, the sufferer re-experiences the event as though it is happening in the current moment. Roméo Dallaire has described the ways that his flashbacks to his time in Rwanda are "digitally clear and often it goes in slow motion, and it comes at different random times. And what it does it is makes you relive the experience. And so for me, the Rwandan genocide—and for my colleagues—isn't 16 years ago. If I sit down and think about it, it happened this morning. I can bring the vividness. I can bring the smell. I can bring that trauma and the sounds back."[46]

While many sufferers have intrusive memories, others may have little or no memory of the trauma event(s). Either way, a person suffering from post-traumatic stress often avoids situations and people that might trigger memories or sensations associated with his/her trauma and distress; however, a person is often unable to predict memory triggers, which leads to increasingly avoidant behavior, often accompanied by disengagement with the outside world and difficulties with intimacy. Sufferers also experience increased arousal, which can include problems falling and/or staying asleep, inability to concentrate, irritability and eruptions of intense anger and hypervigilance. When they return home from service, some veterans describe no longer feeling safe or an overwhelming sense that they no longer fit into society. In public places, many veterans who suffer from hypervigiliance will keep their back to a wall in order to have a clear view of the room, and to keep track of the people who come and go—although many often avoid such busy places altogether.

Sleep disturbances and anxiety/distressing dreams are especially common for people suffering from post-traumatic stress; these tend to continue over the long term for chronic sufferers.[47] Studies with US combat veterans from World War II have shown that while symptoms such as flashbacks and nightmares tend to decrease or disappear over time, sleep disturbances, anxiety and sensations of estrangement often remain.[48] In the film *War in the Mind*, a veteran who performed reconnaissance during World War II described how, for the last 60 years, he had woken up every morning at 4:00 AM with the sensation that he was somewhere he shouldn't be—and that he was back in the war and crawling around in the dark.

In LGen Dallaire's experience, he described how, for post-traumatic stress sufferers, medication and therapy can act in similar ways to a prosthesis for someone who has lost a limb. "The viciousness of this injury, however, is that every now and again something takes away your prosthesis—a sound or something—and you are found helpless. When you have a physical prosthesis you decide when you don't need it anymore…but with PTSD…your defensive mechanisms disappear on you." Dallaire has continued to bring public attention to post-traumatic stress since he believes this is one of the best ways to change the military's attitude and capacities for supporting veterans.[49]

Brigadier General Richard Giguere, who spent 18 months in Afghanistan as Deputy Commander of the Canadian Task Force, has commented that many veterans suffering from post-traumatic stress related to their service in Afghanistan will take time to come forward about their suffering.[50] Many have not sought treatment or compensation due to fears about being stigmatized by fellow military officers, veterans and the public as weak, crazy or malingerers. For example, LCol Chris Linford waited ten years to ask for help. "I thought I was 'fine' and that I could manage my symptoms of anger, hyperarousal, depression, and insomnia. I could not accept that I might be judged as a malingerer or as weak."[51] He also shared a long list of the personal costs to him and his family through his years of post-traumatic suffering and depression: "lack of honesty, loss of self-confidence, loss of my true sense of humour, loss of my identity, hindrance of my ability to be a good husband, father, friend, son, brother, injury to my soul, injury to my relationship with Kathryn and my children, decreased ability to concentrate or to be in crowded places, decreased ability to sleep, profound sadness for extended periods of time, lack of trust in others, loss of patience and understanding, and hopelessness."[52]

As Linford described, the veteran's suffering affects more than just him/herself. Monica Culic, who helped Christian McEachern found the Canadian Veteran Adventure Foundation (see Chapter 4), told me, "It's not just the Forces member that struggles; it's his entire family, it's his kids, it's his wife, it's his best buddy, because when he's great, it's great. And then when he has an episode or is struggling or has flashbacks or he's not sleeping or his medication gets changed or something's triggered him, he's difficult, he manifests all the symptoms, he isolates, he's angry."[53] Author and photographer Penny Coleman, whose ex-husband, a Vietnam veteran suffering from post-traumatic stress, died by suicide, echoed Monica's observation, noting that "living with a PTSD vet is its own traumatic experience."[54] The effects of trauma beyond the primary sufferer are also confirmed by a number of research studies. For example, the Australian Ministry of Veterans Affairs has reported that the children of Vietnam veterans are three times as likely to die by suicide as members of the general population.[55]

While not every person exposed to a traumatic stressor will suffer from post-traumatic stress, those who do will experience symptoms for a long time, even a lifetime.[56] More than three decades after the Korean War, 90–100% of the veterans who were prisoners of war continued to suffer from post-traumatic stress.[57] Today, the mortality rate[58] amongst Vietnam veterans continues to be approximately double that of members of the general public. Vietnam veterans with post-traumatic stress are also more likely to die prematurely compared with veterans not suffering post-traumatic symptoms. Causes of increased early death amongst veterans include both external causes such as suicide, homicide, accidents and substance abuse, but also medical causes such as cardiovascular disease and cancer. The increased mortality rate is thought to be caused by increased substance use, chronic stress and a general lack of self-care amongst Vietnam veterans suffering from continued distress.[59]

Researchers suggest that United Nations peacekeepers also have a high risk of developing symptoms of distress related to both direct and indirect experiences of trauma; however, post-traumatic stress amongst peacekeepers is not well understood, perhaps because each mission varies in intensity and the types of jobs peacekeepers are required to undertake, the circumstances to which soldiers are exposed and how they are able to respond.[60] Souza and colleagues' meta-analysis of 12 studies involving peacekeepers revealed varying levels of distress, from 0.5% to 25.8%.[61] The authors explained that while the general public might perceive the modern peacekeeper's role as less life-threatening and demanding than would occur during war, peacekeepers often face additional burdens. For example, "it is not rare during [a peacekeeping] operation to be attacked by the same population they are supposed to be helping. This kind of threat leads to a situation that is one of the most notable differences between soldiers as warriors and soldiers as peace-keepers: the necessity of upholding restraint."[62]

Peacekeepers often face situations in which there is very little they can do for the population they are charged to protect. In such situations, Shigemura and Nomura observed "while the workers feel powerless-ness, helplessness and anger, they also vicariously experience the vic-tims' feelings of rage, powerlessness and despair, resulting in secondary traumatic stress disorder."[63] The overall prevalence of post-traumatic stress amongst peacekeepers may be underreported because soldiers are concerned about how reporting psychological problems will affect their career, for example fear of being stigmatized and ostracized by peers and superiors.

Trauma and Suicide Amongst Active-Duty Service Members and Veterans

Suffering from post-traumatic experience is also associated with an in-creased risk for attempting suicide.[64] And suicide, reflected LGen Dal-laire, "is the extreme expression of the stress and this injury."[65] Dallaire has been open and honest over the past ten years about his own experi-ences during and following the failed UN mission in Rwanda, including his struggles with substance abuse, cutting and suicide attempts. Once he returned home to Canada from Rwanda, Dallaire couldn't sleep. "I couldn't stand the loudness of silence," he said. And in those moments, he became suicidal; he couldn't live with the pain, and death seemed to be the only option.[66] Nine of Dallaire's comrades from the Rwandan mission have since taken their own lives.[67]

The US has recently seen a drastic increase in suicide amongst ser-vice members. Since the beginning of the war in Afghanistan, more US military personnel have died by suicide than in combat. In 2012, 350 active-duty military personnel took their own lives, a number that, ac-cording to Pentagon reports, rose 22% compared with 2011. This number excludes members of the National Guard and Reserve troops not on active duty when they died by suicide. It also does not include non-fatal suicide attempts amongst military personnel.[68] The reasons for the increase are complex and not fully understood by officials. One study released in May 2013 found that cumulative traumatic brain injuries (TBI) are associated with increased suicide risk. Researchers say that multiple head injuries lead to an increase in psychological symptoms, including depression, thus making suicidal thoughts and behavior more likely.[69] It is estimated that as many as 20% of US military personnel who were stationed in Iraq and Afghanistan suffer from TBI.[70] All of these statistics leave officials expressing deep concern as one million soldiers prepare to leave active service by 2017.

In an August 2013 study published in the *Journal of the American Medical Association*, military researchers asserted that the sharp increase in suicide amongst US military personnel in recent years is not linked to deployment and combat exposure.[71] However, the study has many critics, including Dr. Stephen N. Xenakis, a psychiatrist and a retired Army brigadier general, who told the *New York Times*, "Why would the authors repeatedly insist that there is no association between combat and suicide?... The careful analysis of bad data generates poor evidence."[72] As many of the study's critics point out, deployment is a major factor in operational stress injuries, including post-traumatic stress, depression and drug and alcohol abuse, which are heavily correlated with suicidal thoughts and actions.

The suicide rate amongst the 22 million US veterans is even higher than for serving personnel. The US Department of Veterans Affairs estimates that, in 2010, veteran suicides averaged 22 per day (approximately 8,000 per year), and numbers may be higher since estimates are based on data collected from only 21 states, not including Texas and California, which have large veteran populations.[73] In addition, the study relied on death certificates, and veteran status was unreported or unknown for 23% of all reported suicides.

The Canadian Forces does not keep medical statistics for veterans, nor does it keep information on reservists who have attempted or succeeded in death by suicide. Accordingly, the number of suicides amongst Canadian veterans is unknown.

Suffering Amongst North American Veterans

In both the US and Canada, estimates for the number of soldiers and veterans affected by post-traumatic stress vary widely. Military officials and researchers tend to report lower numbers than experts and veterans' groups outside the military. In a 2013 *TIME Magazine* article, journalist Joe Klein suggested that post-traumatic stress "may affect as many as 40% of the [US] veterans returning from Iraq and Afghanistan."[74]

In Canada, there has been a 47% increase since 2008 in the number of veterans, soldiers and Royal Canadian Mounted Police (RCMP) receiving mental-health-related disability benefits.[75] A 2013 study by the Canadian Department of National Defense (DND) suggested that 13.5% of soldiers who served in Afghanistan from 2001 to 2008 suffer from deployment-related mental injuries.[76] The study's authors acknowledged limitations, since they were able to capture "only diagnoses made by the Canadian Forces mental health services during the follow-up period. We could not identify personnel who had mental disorders that resolved without care; those who were seen only in primary care or outside of the Canadian Forces; those who had not yet fallen ill or had not yet sought care; and those who sought care only after release from the Canadian Forces."[77] Some experts outside the DND have argued that this study severely underestimates the number of soldiers and veterans suffering—and that the real number is likely double that presented by DND researchers.[78] Indeed, Canadian post-deployment screening reports have found that one in four soldiers returning from Afghanistan engages in high-risk drinking or has other experiences ranging from depression to thoughts of suicide.[79] In addition, an increase in domestic violence on Canadian military bases is being attributed to soldiers returning home with physical and psychological injuries.[80] And still other soldiers and veterans may not be suffering from traumatic experiences or brain injuries, but nevertheless feel changed by their military service and are experiencing stress reactions they don't understand.

Compared to their male counterparts, female service members often suffer different traumas while in the military and different challenges when they are released. While women comprise about 15% of the US military, the US Department of Veterans Affairs estimates that as many as 20–30% of serving female soldiers have experienced some form of military sexual trauma (MST), ranging from sexual harassment to sexual assault.[81] Many instances of MST are never reported. In 2012, a survey sponsored by the US Department of Defense (DoD) revealed that, during the previous 12 months, 1.2% of active duty male service members were victims of unwanted sexual contact (USC), compared to 6.1% of female service members.[82] According to DoD estimates, "there may have been approximately 26,000 service members who experienced some form of USC in the year prior to being surveyed."[83] This means that approximately 12,000 serving women and 14,000 serving men were sexually assaulted in the previous year.

Coping with Post-Traumatic Stress

In the spring of 2013, a journalist approached me about my research with veterans who find relief from their post-traumatic symptoms through farming and outdoor activities. She asked a simple question: "Why does it work?" And she likely wanted a quick and clean answer—as though I have perhaps stumbled upon the panacea that society has been looking for to support veterans and soldiers in healing from the wounds of war and military experience.

I suspect that she was disappointed by my answer: that there is no clean cookie-cutter answer for why this works. There are many different interpretations and explanations as to what might be happening. Moreover, many veterans have found healing and relief, and learned to manage their symptoms and move their lives forward, through other avenues. Indeed, most veterans describe multiple avenues of healing, ranging from medication and individual and group therapy to veteran activism and participation in writing groups. Michael Wong wrote, "Healing is a never-ending process, and together we continue to find new insights and deeper levels of healing. Through our pain and anger, our understanding and joy, the skills of writing, speaking, and deep listening have enabled members of the Veteran Writers Group to become a transformative resource for many people and a model for engaging creative expression to help the trauma of war heal."[84] Others find meditation helpful, ranging from secular approaches, such as Mindfulness-Based Stress Reduction based on the work of Dr. Jon Kabat-Zinn, to those aligned with a more spiritual approach and teachings. And still others find relief through art, music, physical activity and exercise, or simply spending time with other veterans.

In June 2013, the cover story of *TIME Magazine*, titled "Can Service Save Us?", described how US veterans are finding public service to be a therapeutic influence in their lives.[85] Similarly, I had a conversation with Col Chuck Hamel of the Canadian Forces, who described at length how volunteering has been important in his own recovery from post-traumatic stress. He also emphasized the importance of the role-play and reenactment approaches offered through the Veterans' Transition Program, a non-profit organization, which has been very successful in supporting some Canadian veterans' transition to civilian life. The program is receiving accolades for its therapeutic approach that has seen depression rates dropping to minimal or no depression at all amongst participants, which the program director has said "helps undo the wiring that military training has implanted in their brain."[86]

Scott Maxwell is executive director of Wounded Warriors Canada, which supports a number of different programs for wounded veterans. During our conversation together, he insisted it was important that veterans' programs be diverse. "Everybody needs help in different ways," said Scott. "There's a fallacy somehow that you're only going to get help if you're talking to a psychiatrist. Of course, psychiatrists can play an instrumental role in these things, but that's not the end-all. There are other ways you can get people to heal."[87]

So while there is no simple answer to the question of why nature contact works, there are some things that have become clear over the course of researching and writing this book. Most studies about the human-nature relationship point to nature contact as improving both self-esteem and mood, and facilitating a sense of social connection and belonging.[88] Many of these aspects are apparent in the veterans' stories. For example, the veterans emphasize teamwork and doing outdoor activities with other veterans, which provide social support and camaraderie with those who have had similar experiences, and give veterans an awareness of once again belonging to a team or family. They also describe the accomplishment and feeling of safety they get from these activities. In addition, there's the importance of meaningful service, which veterans not only get from growing food for other people, but also from serving other vets. Some find meaning in nurturing new life and in feeding other people, as well as in spending time with animals. Nature contact also brings about a sense of being present in the moment, and many veterans describe the peace that comes with that.

Neuroscientists have discovered that drug and alcohol addiction is more likely for those living in social isolation, compared to those living in an enriched environment with stimulating social interactions.[89] Unfortunately, veterans and others suffering from post-traumatic stress tend to fall into patterns of self-medicating with drugs and alcohol while also experiencing social isolation. I have heard many stories of people who suffer alone in their basements, or in their houses with the curtains drawn. Nature, by contrast, provides social lubrication; the veterans whose stories are shared in this book report that it's often easier to connect with other people when fishing, hiking, grooming horses or farming together.

Psychiatrist Jonathan Shay who works with Vietnam veterans echoes the importance of social contact and community, particularly in working through grief. Shay believes that "thwarted, uncommunalized grief is one important reason there are so many long-term psychological casualties of the Vietnam War."[90] Shay acknowledged that the battlefield is not the place for griefwork, but he actively encourages that griefwork be incorporated into military units once soldiers have exited a combat situation. In an interview that aired on PBS, Shay further emphasized the importance of community in veterans' recovery: "Recovery happens only in community," he said. "Peers are the key to recovery." In addition, he argued that "credentialed mental health professionals like me have no place in center stage. It's the veterans themselves, healing each other, that belong at center stage. We are stagehands: get the lights on, sweep out the gum wrappers, count the chairs, make sure it's a safe and warm enough place."[91]

◈ ◈ ◈

In the chapters that follow, veterans' lives and experiences do exhibit patterns that often include isolation, avoidance and anger. Yet their stories suggest another approach to healing and recovery that they each came to on their own: spending time connecting with nature, ranging from hiking and canoeing to farming, gardening and interacting with animals. While most of the veterans find that their nature experiences are important in combination with other forms of treatment, they all emphasize that nature contact has been crucial in supporting their efforts to cope with their injuries and moving toward a place of recovery.

2

Connections between Nature and Healing

Humans have a long history of turning to nature to ease what ails us. There is now a substantial body of empirical research on the interconnections between human health and nature—which includes both animals and the wider world around us. Much of the research suggests that increased contact with nature (as compared to a human-built environment) is important at physical, psychological, cognitive and emotional levels. To put it another way, nature seems essential to our sense of being human.

Academic theories and research studying the human-nature relationship are diverse, but tend to be connected by an agreement that the human brain evolved in complex environments, in which our survival depended on constant interaction with other creatures and the Earth. Humans today, despite our technological prowess and increasingly urban lifestyles, are genetically identical to our hunter-gatherer ancestors who evolved in concert with all the other plants and creatures on this planet. Most researchers assert that, while often repressed in modern times and culture, deep ecological instincts continue to be rooted in the human psyche.

Despite the growing number of empirical studies about the benefit of nature-based activity, a common challenge experienced by veterans' groups is that, regardless of many anecdotal reports that nature-based activities are helping veterans, there's little money available from funders because very few studies have focused on veterans. This is starting to change (veteran-specific research is described at the end of this chapter), but many of the results from other research can also apply to veteran populations. Accordingly, this chapter explores many different studies and approaches to understanding the human-nature relationship.

Historical Connections

Incorporating nature into human healing and rehabilitation is not a novel idea. Social historian Theodore Roszak observed that, at one time, "all psychologies were 'ecopsychologies.' Those who sought to heal the soul took it for granted that human nature is densely embedded in the world we share with animal, vegetable, mineral, and all the unseen powers of the cosmos."[1] Connections between nature experiences and human health have been accepted by poets, sages and indigenous peoples, amongst others, for thousands of years. Ancient Greek healing places and temples were purposefully located on hilltops in the countryside with views of the ocean, around the same time that Taoists in China were building greenhouses and cultivating gardens as part of their approaches to maintain health and well-being.[2] Chinese mystics often escaped the activity and clamor of towns for the countryside, where they sought to find and restore their souls, while the Christian Bible tells numerous stories of devotees who retreated to the desert to have contact with God.[3]

In the European Middle Ages, gardens were deemed an important facet of human healing, particularly in monastic communities. With its centrally located water feature and its open view of the sky, the traditional monastery cloister was designed to facilitate meditation for both resident monks and patients.[4] During the Victorian era, gardens were often found in hospitals.[5] Beginning in the nineteenth century, French churches advocated community gardens as a way to improve the circumstances of the working poor.[6] Meanwhile, in the US, the Quakers' Friends Hospital in Pennsylvania treated patients suffering from mental ill health with gardening and walks in surrounding lands.[7]

In the 1960s, psychoanalyst Harold Searles argued that most studies in psychoanalysis considered nature to be irrelevant, "as though human life were lived out in a vacuum—as though the human race were alone in the universe."[8] In response, and drawing on his work with schizo-phrenic patients, Searles began articulating his vision that nature is of primary importance to the human psyche, since the prevailing condi-tions in which the human personality matures comprises "predomi-nantly nonhuman elements—trees, clouds, stars, landscapes, buildings, and so on ad infinitum."[9] Searles observed that when humans ignore the connections between their psyche and nature, it endangers their psy-chological well-being, and in his later work, he maintained that "an eco-logically healthy relatedness to our nonhuman environment is essential to the development and maintenance of our sense of being human."[10] Today, however, human health is primarily understood within the urban-industrial context of the individual human being, wherein phar-macology, psychology and psychiatry are presented as the best meth-ods for supporting struggling individuals, while relationships within the wider world of nature are thought to be irrelevant.

The importance of the human-nature relationship is beginning to gain attention once more. A wide range of empirical studies have been conducted in the past 20 years to explore the physiological and emo-tional benefits of natural settings, as well as the ways nature contributes to and enhances humans' attention spans, and how regular experiences in nature seem to result in better mental health.[11] Thirty years ago in the prominent research journal *Science*, Roger Ulrich described his dis-covery that hospital patients recovering from gall bladder surgery who had a view of trees from their hospital beds required a shorter stay and fewer medications, and experienced fewer postsurgical complications, than patients whose windows looked onto a brick wall.[12] A parallel study found that prison inmates with a view of farm fields used prison health care services less often than those who looked onto an inner courtyard.[13] Research in workplace settings has demonstrated a similar pattern, where employees whose window provides a view of trees or a park are sick less often as well as more satisfied with their jobs compared to peers without such a view.[14] It seems, too, that even pictures of na-ture can positively influence people's moods and concentration.[15] And when asked to identify the most significant place during their child-hood, nearly all adults in Rachel Sebba's study (96.5%) described a place outdoors, from parks and seashores to farms and other rural areas.[16] Based on such findings, some practitioners have begun to incorporate nature into a variety of therapy settings, including treatment for brain injuries and neurological illness, personality disorders and attention deficit hyperactivity disorder.[17]

Nature, Restoration and Stress Recovery

One area of growing academic scholarship focuses specifically on nature and restoration (also referred to as stress recovery). When humans are tired and stressed and our energies are depleted, we can experience dark moods, heightened arousal in the autonomic nervous system and diminished capacities for focused attention. Restoration, then, refers to renewing these diminished resources and faculties, to enhancing mood, decreasing arousal and regaining the ability to focus attention on specific activities.

Two experiments by Terry Hartig's research team in Sweden compared the emotional and physiological effects of natural and urban settings. First, the researchers tested participants while sitting either in a room with a view of trees or a room with no window; they found that blood pressure decreased for the people in the room with the view, but increased for those in the room with no window. Next, they took participants walking, in either a nature reserve or a medium-density housing development. The participants who walked in the nature reserve experienced a decrease in blood pressure and reported a decline in feelings of anger and aggression, while those who walked in the urban setting experienced an increase in all three areas.[18] Researchers at the University of Essex conducted a similar study, comparing the effects of an outdoor walk in the woods and an indoor walk at a shopping mall on participants' self-esteem, depression and tension. They found that the outdoor walk often improved all three emotions.[19] Thus, like getting regular sleep, it is suggested that "regular access to restorative [natural] environments can interrupt processes that negatively affect health and well-being in the short- and long-term."[20]

Researchers in Scotland conducted two parallel studies—this time with adults from different health groups. The first investigated the outcomes of a walk in a rural setting on adults with good and poor mental health. Prior to the walk, the adults in the good health group reported overall better mood and self-esteem as well as lower stress levels than those struggling with mental illness. In their post-walk survey, researchers found that the walk had improved the mood and lowered the stress of people in both groups, but that those with poor mental health reported more benefit. The second study took the same participants on two walks, this time one urban walk and one rural walk. The participants with good mental health reported mood and stress benefits from the rural walk, but no difference from the urban walk. However, both walks contributed to positive change in the moods of adults with poor mental health, although there were again more benefits from the rural walk.[21]

In another experiment, Terry Hartig and Henk Staats tested participants' preference for walking in the city or in a forest, and found that the more fatigued participants were, the more likely they were to express a preference for walking in a forest.[22] Another longitudinal study uncovered a positive correlation between cold summer weather in Sweden and the levels of antidepressants prescribed by doctors. The researchers hypothesized that in summers with cool rainy weather, Swedes were less likely to spend time outdoors and therefore did not benefit from the restorative properties of nature, thus leading to increased levels of depression.[23] Meanwhile, a Danish longitudinal study involving civil servants in the City of Århus, Denmark, who work in indoor compared with outdoor environments during the winter months, discovered that outdoor work offered some protection against mood difficulties.[24]

In another comprehensive study involving more than 10,000 adult Danes, a group of researchers examined the relationships between participants' levels of stress and health-related quality of life, and the proximity of their homes to green space. The study found that those living within one kilometer of green space tended to report better health and health-related quality of life than those living further away. Moreover, the more often participants visited those green spaces, the less stress they reported. Meanwhile, respondents living more than one kilometer away from green space had a higher probability of experiencing stress.[25]

A study in Taiwan showed that the presence of plants in a junior-high classroom positively influenced students' behavior and well-being. In particular, students in the classroom with plants tended to rate themselves both as more comfortable in the classroom and as feeling more friendly toward others than students in a classroom without plants.[26] Meanwhile, researchers at the University of Twente in the Netherlands suggested that indoor plants in hospital rooms can reduce patients' feelings of stress, although they admitted the effects might have more to do with the "perceived attractiveness of the hospital room" than interaction with the plants themselves.[27]

Some researchers propose that even nature experiences of short duration are worthwhile. David Cole and Troy Hall examined whether the amount of time spent in a wilderness environment was important to individuals' experience of restoration as well as whether the number of people encountered along a trail affected hikers' experiences. They found that no matter the trail congestion or the length of time, most participants reported substantial "stress reduction and mental rejuvenation." Cole and Hall concluded that the restorative effects of spending time in nature can occur in a relatively short amount of time, and whether one is alone or in the company of others.[28]

Researchers studying stress recovery propose that the importance of nature in human life stems from the fact that the human brain co-evolved with other creatures and with rivers, oceans, rocks, deserts, winds, skies, trees and plants. While over the years humanity has experienced high rates of cultural and technological change, the rate of biological evolution has been quite slow, which means that human nervous systems today are virtually the same as those of our long-ago ancestors. Indeed, the role of nature in renewing humans' ability to concentrate is considered by many scientists to be an evolutionary adaptation. Stephen Kaplan argued that natural settings require a reduced amount of energy and effort compared with urban settings, and the human body is thought to respond instinctively to nature in a way that it cannot to the built environment. The type of constant linear attention to a specific task often required in our schooling and jobs today would have been dangerous, even deadly, for our ancestors, since they could have been easily surprised by predators. Instead of focusing for a long time on any one thing, our ancestors needed to be constantly aware of their surroundings and to frequently shift their awareness.[29]

Accordingly, some researchers have suggested that nature requires a different type of attention than human-built environments, leading it to play a restorative function for human attention.[30] Others have argued that nature provides biological support for recovery from stress.[31] No matter the explanation, however, the recent research shows that spending time in nature is genuinely important for human beings.[32]

Wilderness (Adventure) Therapy and Wilderness Experiences

Throughout the 20th century, there were anecdotal accounts of the benefits of "camping therapy" in North America.[33] Indeed, wilderness therapy has gained increased attention as an approach to experiential therapy that combines cognitive therapy and/or humanistic therapy within a nature setting typically far away from urban contexts.[34] Advocates argue that wilderness therapy, which involves programs offered by a licensed therapist and trained clinical staff and a treatment plan for each participant, must be clearly differentiated from improvements in well-being that people experience as a consequence or side effect of spending time in nature.[35]

The major studies in wilderness therapy have reported improved self-esteem and sense of social connection as well as interpersonal development and enhanced social skills.[36] Many wilderness therapy programs have concentrated on treating young people living in psychiatric environments as well as those with eating disorders, emotional and/or substance abuse problems. The central focus of such therapies involves an element of perceived risk, in which participants are challenged to "experience something new, or to experience themselves in a new situation."[37] In addition, all participants are challenged as a team, which means they need to rely on and trust one another to successfully complete tasks and activities.

Toward the end of the 20th century, there were more than 700 wilderness experience programs in the US alone, and those programs specifically designed as wilderness therapeutic interventions numbered somewhere from 60 to 100.[38] In Robert Greenway's 22 years of running a wilderness therapy training program at Sonoma State University, he became a deep believer in the power of nature to facilitate changed psychological processes. From his experience, he has suggested that a wilderness encounter needs to last ten or more days in order to promote meaningful and lasting change.[39]

Studies with Children and Older Adults

Studies with both children and older adults are pointing to the importance of nature throughout a person's life cycle. James Sallis, program director for the Active Living Research Program for the Robert Wood Johnson Foundation, told Richard Louv that children with indoor, inactive upbringings are more likely to experience struggles with mental health and well-being.[40] And researchers Andrea Faber Taylor and Frances Kuo assert that there is enough evidence from numerous studies of the relationships between children and nature to support the notion that nature is crucial for children's cognitive, social and psychological development.[41] Elsewhere, Taylor, Kuo and Sullivan have suggested that natural environments can support children with attention-deficit hyperactivity disorder (ADHD). In focus groups with parents, they discovered that urban environments and modern technologies often aggravate a child's ADHD symptoms, but natural settings never exacerbate—and often alleviate—the symptoms. One parent shared that a Disneyland trip was too stimulating for her child, but a camping trip to a state park resulted in a vacation the whole family enjoyed because her child was relaxed, happy and calm. Another parent described how his son's struggles with ADHD were minimal when he was engaged in outdoor activities such as hitting golf balls or fishing. The researchers also discovered that the ADHD symptoms of children who tend to play in indoor settings such as basements with few or no windows were more severe than for children who played outdoors.[42]

A teacher friend told me about a child in her elementary school classroom who was diagnosed with severe ADHD. One day, as she was trying to get a sense of how best to work with this child and create a positive school experience for him, she asked, "Where do you feel best?" He confidently replied, "When I am in nature." This child did not need a study to know when and where he felt well in the world.

Canadian researchers in Toronto recently studied children whose school grounds incorporate diverse aspects of nature settings, such as food, wildflower and/or butterfly gardens, ponds and trees. The children in these play settings were more physically active and had a better understanding of nutrition and where their food comes from (compared with children who played on the conventional asphalt and turf spaces found at most schools). And perhaps more importantly, the children with the green school grounds showed tremendous increases in civil behavior and cooperative, collaborative and respectful play; they were much more likely to demonstrate increased curiosity and wonder about the world, as well as to think more creatively. The children who played in natural spaces were also more likely to integrate groups traditionally excluded from their play, and to overlook the habitual divisions of gender, socioeconomic status, physical ability and ethnicity, so that all children played together.[43]

A longitudinal study with children from low-income urban families suggested that "the natural environment may play a far more significant role in [their] well-being...than has previously been recognized."[44] At the beginning of the study, all families resided in substandard, low-income housing. Then, through Habitat for Humanity's self-help housing program, the families relocated to better housing with improved access to nature. Over time, researchers saw a marked improvement in the children's cognitive functioning. The study's author, Nancy Wells, noted that the more access to nature the children had, the more they seemed to benefit from moving to their new home. Wells also pointed to a study by Swedish researchers that examined two different daycare settings, one of which was the more typical urban variety (with a playground area surrounded by low plants, a cycling path and tall buildings) while the other featured an "old mature orchard surrounded by pasture on two sides, woodland on the third, and a wild, overgrown garden with tall trees and large rocks next to the building."[45] At this second daycare, children played outside for a substantial amount of time every day, and the researchers reported that compared to the standard daycare, children at the "more natural day care center had greater attentional capacity."[46]

At the other end of the age spectrum, Mooney and Nicell followed patients with Alzheimer's disease at five different care facilities for two years. Two of the care facilities provided patients with access to gardens, while at the other three, patients had no access to nature settings. Over the two years, violent assaults by Alzheimer's patients at the three facilities with no access to gardens increased significantly (violence is a common occurrence amongst Alzheimer's patients because the disease causes a person's cognitive processes to deteriorate over time). Meanwhile, at the two facilities with gardens, levels of violence stayed the same or even decreased slightly when patients were given regular access to the gardens.[47]

Susan Rodiek's study with elderly nursing home residents also showed a number of positive results for residents who spent time in a garden setting, many of whom reported significantly lower levels of anxiety and positive mood compared with those who spent time only indoors. Measurements of the residents' cortisol (a stress hormone) levels confirmed these findings, where the cortisol levels of garden participants were reduced by two and a half times those of the study's indoor participants.[48]

In 2012, the Goldielea Care and Nursing Home in Scotland launched a birdwatching program for its residents. The care home's activities coordinator, Carol Wilkie, reported that the staff soon began to notice increased social interaction amongst the birdwatchers. And residents themselves reported an increased sense of social inclusion and connectedness.[49] Meanwhile, Swedish researchers conducted a study amongst persons with early-stage dementia and found that outdoor activities provided sensory experiences, social interactions, a sense of freedom and independence and self-confidence that were important to patients suffering from early dementia. Most importantly, patients described "being outdoors as a confirmation of the self."[50]

Stimulating Our Senses

Landscape designer C. Colston Burrell has pointed to the power of gardens to stimulate the human senses of sight, sound, touch and smell. He has argued that scent is perhaps the most powerful aspect in a garden, noting that while fragrances' effects on human beings are not fully understood, they are known to have psychological, physiological and neurological benefits and to change hormone production and brain chemistry. Even at undetectable levels, odors can influence the central nervous system. Indeed, this is the premise behind aromatherapy as part of alternative or complementary medicine practices. Some scientists hypothesize that the capacity of fragrances to affect us in these diverse ways derives from the human nasal passages' direct connection to the brain's center for emotions and memory.[51] In their research on cut flower arrangements and lavender fragrance, researchers at Kansas State University concluded that sight and smell play important roles in reducing stress and producing positive emotional responses in college students.[52]

Horticulture therapist Elizabeth Messer Diehl has further suggested that interacting with plants is a powerful method for reawakening and stimulating the senses through fragrance, color, texture, taste and sound. The ways that a garden can completely engage a person's corporeal experience have physical, emotional and cognitive benefits. As a person embraces the experience, Messer Diehl suggested it becomes possible to connect more deeply to the garden, thus further enhancing and bringing forth the healing properties of nature. Additionally, she reflected on the power of particular scents to "stimulate bodily organs to release neurochemicals that help eliminate pain, induce sleep, and create a sense of well-being."[53]

Botanist, medical and agricultural researcher Diana Beresford-Kroeger reflected that taking a summer walk in a mature pine forest has, for thousands of years, been considered to be good for a person's health. Bringing attention to the biochemical properties in plants, she noted that "the fresh leaves [in a pine forest] exert a stimulant effect on breathing with the addition of mild anaesthetic properties. There is possibly some mild narcotic function also in pines." Further, the sound of winds blowing through pine boughs has been found to soothe people suffering from illness. Beresford-Kroeger's work points to similar benefits provided by other trees to both humans and the wider planetary community.[54] Indeed, viewed from the context of her research, the emotional and physiological benefits that occur when people spend time in nature are quite possibly influenced by the medicinal properties released by the plants and trees around them.

Biophilia and Ecological Intelligence

There are many theories about why nature is important to the human psyche. For example, the term *biophilia* was first suggested by psychologist Erich Fromm in the 1960s. Bio- comes from the Greek *bio*, meaning "one's life" but more generally referring to anything living or alive, and -philia from the Greek *philia*, meaning "affection" and stemming from *philos*, "love," so that biophilia quite literally means "love of life." Fromm suggested biophilia as a term to refer to orientations toward self-preservation or the life drive. He contrasted this term with necrophilia, which he suggested was the opposite human attraction and orientation toward death and destructive behavior as well as qualities of greed and self-absorption.[55] Later, renowned biologist E. O. Wilson expanded the notion of biophilia to encompass the love of all life forms. Wilson has observed that human beings have an affinity for all life, which expresses a deep-rooted genetic and biological need. He believes that humanity itself is defined by our interactions and kinship with other organisms.[56]

Meanwhile, author and psychologist Daniel Goleman, perhaps best known for his work on emotional intelligence that draws on Howard Gardner's theory of multiple intelligences, has promoted what he calls ecological intelligence: "our ability to adapt to our ecological niche."[57] Goleman suggested that ecological intelligence is a receptivity and empathetic responsiveness for all life. He has argued that we need to stop setting ourselves apart from nature, instead to remember and acknowledge that human life is inextricable from the ecosystems we inhabit and that all organisms mutually impact and affect one another, in ways that are either beneficial or harmful.

Insights from Ecopsychology

Andy Fisher, a leading scholar in the field of ecopsychology as well as a psychotherapist in private practice in Eastern Ontario, offers a different perspective. The purpose of ecopsychology is to "place all psychological and spiritual matters within the context of our membership in the natural world."[58] Ecopsychology works to locate the human psyche within the wider world, to show that our psyche is never separate from the world.[59] Indeed, ecopsychologists regard urban-industrial society to be at the root of much of the suffering (grief, despair and anxiety) in modern times, since our culture dismisses ecological instincts deeply rooted in the human psyche, or what some refer to as the "ecological unconscious." The most important contribution of ecopsychology to *Field Exercises* is perhaps its primary assertion that "genuine sanity is grounded in the reality of the natural world."[60]

Fisher warns about the language that often accompanies the empirical research reviewed in this chapter: it continues to maintain human/nature divisions and sees nature as a psychological resource.[61] In my conversation with him, Fisher expanded on this idea. While research points to deep interconnections between humans and nature, Fisher believes it is limited and "just the tip of the iceberg." Fisher told me that the modern world confines our perceptions and sensory abilities in ways that make it difficult to understand or bring meaning to nature experiences "beyond the obviousness of them when we're having them." He is hopeful that as more people recognize the importance of nature contact, better ways will come to speak about these experiences as integral to our lives.

After an experience of trauma, Fisher observed, both the body and the psyche need to regain their sense of security. And the body is capable of recognizing when it is in the presence of what it needs, or what it's implying. "If I'm hungry, then my body's implying food," Fisher explained. "And if I'm traumatized, my body's going to be implying certain experiences that will help restore a sense of security or calm or peace or life." In particular, Andy Fisher reflected that when veterans describe how their nature experiences support their recovery, this suggests that what is being called for—what their bodies are implying—is vitality and an experience in the world of nature to carry life forward. It is through our bodies that we have access to nature; indeed, it is through our bodies that we are nature. "In order to complete these trauma experiences, or recover from the trauma experiences," said Fisher, "[when the veteran] comes across the river, [he has a] shift in his experience. His body is saying, 'This is it! This is what I'm implying.' So that takes our thinking of the healing process beyond the therapy office into a more-than-human field of what might be called for in the healing process."

Fisher also described how ecology is the study of relationships between an organism and its environment—called an organism-environment field—and that this ecological way of thinking can help in understanding the differences between a therapy room and a natural setting. "We tend to split ourselves from environment rather than understanding the unity of organism and environment, body and world," Fisher said. The therapy room is limited in space, which generally requires a sitting posture. "That really limits the possibilities of healing by thinking in terms of that organism-environment field," Fisher explained. Ecopsychology, meanwhile, asks about other organism-environment fields and shows that natural settings bring possibilities and postures beyond the sitting position required in a therapy room. "It's quite a risk for therapists to step outside the office," Fisher acknowledged, since this is often their comfort zone. But he observed that veterans' experiences in nature demonstrate that other settings are both possible and essential. "The work you're doing with the vets is demonstrating that there are other organism-environment fields that would be important to recognize—for how they perhaps take us to a deeper place in terms of that resonance with the world...that really draws on a very deep memory of our place in the world."[62]

Studies in Neuroscience

Neuroscientist Kelly Lambert, the Macon and Joan Brock Professor and Chair of Psychology at Randolph-Macon College in Virginia, conducts research on stress and coping. In her book *Lifting Depression*, she showed that human bodies, senses and emotions were crucial to human evolution and becoming, but today people all over the world are engaging almost exclusively in cognitive tasks that leave the body behind. And Lambert contended that "the environment around us is a critical variable in determining the severity of our stress responses in different situations."[63]

During my conversation with her, Lambert described a standard neuroscience experiment: placing rats into enriched environments using artificial stimuli (such as plastic toys, tunnels and mirrors) and then testing their cognitive behavior. Some of her students wondered what might happen if they compared these artificially enriched environments to naturally enriched environments. They designed an experiment in which some rats received the standard enriched environment (the "city rats"), while another group received sticks and leaves, small logs and pebbles to move around (the "country rats"). The rats in both settings had the same ability to manipulate everything, and each of the artificial and natural objects served the same purpose, such as a plastic tunnel or a log to hide inside.

When Lambert and her students tested the cognitive behavior of the rats in each setting (how smart they were), there was little difference. However, said Lambert, "We are seeing a difference in emotional resilience. The animals in the natural environment are bolder, and their stress hormones are at a healthier level." She tied this result into the larger picture of urban life and the artificial stimuli that constantly surrounds us humans, which she suggested is causing us to lose "some of our emotional edge," and is resulting in higher rates of depression in urban areas. "Our country rats are a little more emotionally stable," she said.

"If you think about how our brains evolved to be in nature, not in an office building, you are tapping into some of your natural healing resources," Lambert told me. Referring to studies such as Roger Ulrich's research with hospital patients who recovered better with a view of trees, she continued, "Nature does tap into some healing properties, both with the immune system and with emotional resilience. You're becoming a little more emotionally tough or resilient by just being exposed to nature."[64]

Nature's Antidepressant, *M. vaccae*

In 2002, Graham Rook and Laura Brunet, both from the Royal Free and University College Medical School in London, published an article in *The Biologist* called "Give us this day our daily germs." In it, they argued that one of the effects of modern urban lifestyles in wealthy countries is reduced exposure to organisms, such as mycobacteria, that live in soil and water. The researchers contended that this reduced exposure is improperly activating human immune systems, resulting in higher rates of some types of allergy and disease.[65] Indeed, many researchers are now investigating the ways that various bacteria in the world around us activate our immune systems in ways that can protect us physiologically, behaviorally and cognitively.

Of particular interest are studies examining the effects of *Mycobacterium vaccae* (*M. vaccae*), a strain of bacteria commonly found in soil. While testing the effects of heat-killed *M. vaccae* on lung cancer patients receiving chemotherapy, oncologists made an unexpected and important discovery: the bacteria did not seem to affect patients' survival rates, but patients did report an improved quality of life, including better cognitive functioning and a sense of vitality, as well as some relief from both chemotherapy-related symptoms and cancer symptoms.[66]

Neuroscientists at the University of Bristol decided to investigate these findings further, and discovered that heat-killed *M. vaccae* altered emotional behavior in mice. Specifically, the bacteria produced antidepressant-like effects by triggering neurons in the brain to produce serotonin.[67] Serotonin plays many key roles within the bodies of humans and other animals—among them, mood regulation, but also "aggression, appetite, cognition, emesis, endocrine function, gastrointestinal function, motor function, neurotrophism, perception, sensory function, sex, sleep, respiration, and vascular function."[68] Accordingly, antidepressant medications, amongst other drugs, are often designed to affect serotonin levels. Chris Lowry, lead author of the University of Bristol study, noted that such research results in a better understanding of the connections between healthy immune systems and mental health. "They also leave us wondering if we shouldn't all be spending more time playing in the dirt," he said.[69]

Since serotonin supports learning and cognition, Dorothy Matthews and Susan Jenks at The Sage Colleges were interested in whether ingesting live *M. vaccae* would decrease the stress response in mice, while also improving their learning ability. Indeed, their research found this to be the case. When compared with a control group, mice that ingested live *M. vaccae* prior to and during the experiment were able to navigate more quickly through a complex maze—almost twice as fast!—while also demonstrating fewer anxiety-related behaviors. But the *M. vaccae* effects were temporary. Matthews and Jenks tested both groups again after none of the mice had ingested *M. vaccae* for three weeks, and there was no longer a difference in their maze performance and anxiety levels.[70] This research suggests that we require continual interaction with natural environments, during which we ingest or inhale *M. vaccae*, to benefit.

Mental Fatigue and Aggression

Stephen Kaplan found that people whose directed attention is fatigued become irritable and often seek to be alone.[71] And Terry Hartig and colleagues suggest that the ways in which nature can be associated with anger reduction merits special attention.[72] Indeed, a study by Frances Kuo and William Sullivan found a connection between lack of exposure to natural settings and aggression/violence amongst inner-city Chicago residents living in poverty. The authors suggested that the ongoing stress associated with poverty and the pervasive risks of crime and unpredictable violence for people living in poverty-stricken neighborhoods tend to contribute to heightened levels of mental fatigue, since individuals are constantly on guard for signs of trouble. Stress and mental fatigue can increase aggressive behavior. Interestingly, the researchers found significantly lower levels of intrafamily violence amongst families living in public housing apartments that had access to natural environments such as trees and grass immediately outside apartments compared with families whose apartments opened onto barren land or concrete.

Kuo and Sullivan urged caution in extrapolating the results of their study to apply to other settings. They argued that further research is needed to better understand the connections between aggression and mental fatigue, and the influence of nature on reducing aggression.[73] However, one might, for example, draw parallels to soldiers' experiences in combat, wherein soldiers are also under constant stress, hypervigilant for signs of danger and/or situations of concern and often lack access to restorative settings.

Relationships with Animals

The act of caring for animals can help to bring people out of themselves and become more open to the world around them. Some studies have also found that pets reduce feelings of loneliness and social isolation. Researchers Erika Friedmann and Heesook Son, who evaluated many of the empirical studies on human-animal relationships, suggested that "the impact of pet ownership on health seems to be most important for highly stressed or socially isolated individuals."[74] An emerging and growing area in veteran care involves companion animals for men and women who suffer from stress injuries. A number of the veterans featured in this book describe the importance of their relationships with animals, including dogs and horses. Animals keep post-traumatic stress survivors focused on the present moment and provide a reason to get up in the morning; a dog, for example, needs to be fed and taken for a walk.

There have been numerous studies involving human relationships with other animals in recent years, ranging from animals as companions to their effects on blood pressure, stress and minor health problems. For example, a study published in the *American Journal of Cardiology* examined the effects of pet ownership and social support on one-year survival rates after a heart attack. The researchers discovered that heart-attack survivors who were also dog-owners were much less likely to die within one year than those without a dog. Patients who had more social support were also more likely to be alive after one year.[75] Another study concluded that, compared to a control group, patients with acute depression who spent 30 minutes with a dog experienced a significant reduction in levels of anxiety.[76]

Studies have also found that companion animals and animal-assisted therapies are helpful for children, including hospitalized adolescents and children suffering from trauma and post-traumatic stress.[77] Israeli researchers recently determined that, over a period of three months, dog-assisted therapy held significant benefits for teenage girls who had experienced physical or sexual abuse. The girls' symptoms of depression and psychological distress declined considerably, as did their risk for developing post-traumatic stress.[78] Another study that examined pain intervention in children found that children participating in an animal-assisted therapy program experienced a fourfold reduction in levels of pain, compared to a control group. The study's authors explain that "exposure to a pet or other friendly animal induces the release of endorphins, which induce a feeling of well-being, and lymphocytes, which increase the immune response."[79] And researchers in Norway found that a four-month horse program, which incorporated both working with and riding horses, led to an increase in perceived social support for 12- to 15-year-olds without behavioral problems.[80]

The number of equine-assisted therapy programs with a broad client base in Canada and the US is growing. For example, participants in a US-based equine therapy study demonstrated significant improvements in well-being, including a decrease in psychological distress. Participants also reported being "(a) more oriented in the present; (b) better able to live more fully in the here-and-now; (c) less burdened by regrets, guilt, and resentments; (d) less focused on fears related to the future; (e) more independent; and (f) more self-supportive."[81]

A 2012 report by the Canadian Agency for Drugs and Technologies in Health found that both dog- and horse-assisted therapies can contribute to short-term improvements in "mental health function and socialization in patients with depression, trauma, schizophrenia, and dementia." The Agency recommended more longitudinal studies to better understand the long-term benefits of interacting with dogs and horses for these patient groups.[82] In 2013, Veterans Affairs Canada provided funding to Can Praxis to study the effectiveness of equine-assisted therapy for veterans (see Chapter 7).[83]

Researchers in Norway have also suggested that working with and caring for farm animals provides another animal-assisted activity to enhance mental, social and physical health, with benefits that include decreased levels of anxiety, decreased depression, increased self-esteem, self-worth and self-confidence. Even sense of joy, positive influences on coping ability and new-found social connections increased.[84] Another Norwegian study found that, compared with a control group, participants suffering from clinical depression who worked with dairy cattle twice weekly for 12 weeks experienced a significant decrease in their levels depression and anxiety, and an increase in their sense of self-efficacy.[85] These gains were maintained during the three-month period after the intervention. It was especially important for participants to feel challenged by complex tasks, such as milking, feeding, cleaning and moving cows, as well as interacting with the farmer. Participants did not seem to benefit when engaged only in beginner tasks, such as mucking and grooming.[86]

Research with Veterans and Nature

Despite the historical connections between veterans, gardening and farming mentioned in the introduction, only now are some doctors, psychiatrists, psychologists and other caregivers realizing that nature contact can support the transition to civilian life and ease suffering from military stress and trauma. For example, Dr. Marnie Burkman, a psychiatrist who works with veterans in Colorado, has observed in her own practice "the powerful effect that nature has to promote healing."[87]

In June 2013, researchers at the University of Michigan published the results of their study with the Sierra Club demonstrating that veterans who participated in multi-day camping and hiking trips reported an improved sense of mental well-being, as well as feeling less socially isolated. Many of the veterans continued to experience an improved sense of well-being a month after the excursion, and those who were suffering the most seemed to report the most improvement.[88] The year 2013 also saw the publication of *War Trauma and Its Wake: Expanding the Circle of Healing*, which features two chapters that bring attention to the benefits of outdoor programs for veterans. One chapter includes a clinical vignette about the Canadian Veteran Adventure Foundation (CVAF).[89] The chapter's authors, a psychologist and psychiatrist who both work with veterans, were "profoundly moved" during a weekend trip with the CVAF, when they observed how "smiles and laughter replaced [veterans'] anxiety and fear."[90] The chapter also includes insights from two participants who said that the weekend trip was "the first major positive experience for so many of us in years."[91] The other chapter, by Lt. Col. Valvincent Reyes, examined outdoor therapy approaches in the US. Reyes contended that outdoor activities are especially relevant for active-duty soldiers and veterans, since much of their military training also took place outdoors.[92]

Another anthology, *Greening in the Red Zone: Disaster, Resilience and Community Greening*, explores how people around the world are "turning to nature in time of disaster or crisis."[93] One of the editors, Keith Tidball, a former National Guard infantry officer, has been conducting research with veterans for a number of years. In 2012, he hosted a Returning Warriors Fall Workshop at the 4H Camp Wabasso in Jefferson County, New York, to solicit recommendations for supporting wounded veterans and their families through outdoor recreation and nature-based activities, and to investigate what role environmental educators might play in this work.[94] Tidball's current research focuses on the benefits of hunting and fishing for veterans' reintegration. During a conversation with me, he described three layers of benefits that accrue when veterans become involved in these activities: 1) the self-confidence from realizing they can be successful at something, and the "social benefit of being around the campfire and sharing mutual interest" with other veterans; 2) the benefits of "urgent biophilia"; and 3) "a reawakening or rekindling of a sense of ecological identity," a sense of being part of the larger world, which often leads veterans to become involved in other projects. Tidball also told me that recreation groups for veterans replicate many of the positive aspects of a military environment, including "objectives and mission orientation, and camaraderie."

One of the biggest challenges to getting more veterans involved in hunting and fishing activities, Tidball said, is a public perception and attitudinal barrier. Many people become upset by the idea that combat soldiers are going into the woods with guns. When he described his encounters with this perception, Tidball could not hide his irritation and disbelief. Most veterans, he said, do fine with such activities. "And those that aren't, or are afraid they might not be, wouldn't be participating in these activities." The military and the US Veterans Administration also seem resistant to hunting and fishing, in part Tidball suspects, because "they have some of those same sorts of stereotypes.... Those aren't the things they want to be seen as publically supporting in terms of their veterans' programming, even though there are lots of vets asking for it." At the same time, within the military community, there's also resistance to gardening, which can be seen as too "frou-frou," despite the fact, Tidball said, that "many hardcore front-of-the-battle-area warrior types get a lot of benefit out of gardening."

A further benefit of hunting and fishing, particularly for veterans for whom combat has been confusing, Tidball said, is that it can support them in bringing new understanding to and making meaning of death. "The inability to make sense of killing in combat is one of the characteristics of war," Tidball explained. "And there's a whole gambit of emotions that someone might go through when they've shot a deer, and they go up to it, and confront what has been troubling [them] in terms of what death means. And in many cases, there's a very beautiful resolution to those problems because they're able to bring meaning back to the taking of life, including their own nourishment."[95]

Another study was completed by researchers from East Carolina University in conjunction with the non-profit organization Keeping Warriors Outdoors. Over the course of a four-day retreat, researchers found that military personnel who participated developed a comfort zone through social relationships and bonds, and many felt able to try new activities and to connect with others.[96] These findings echo a 1996 study of a five-day Outward Bound experience involving Vietnam veterans suffering from combat-related PTSD. That study involved 219 veterans from two different VA Medical Centers. Half the veterans were assigned to a control group, while the other half participated in Outward Bound activities, including three days of climbing, camping, hiking, white water rafting and/or navigating rope courses. The study concluded that the Outward Bound experience did not have much effect on specific PTSD symptoms, measured according to a standardized medical scale in terms of intrusions, avoidance and arousal patterns.

(In many ways, these results are not surprising. To expect that a three-day outdoor experience would reduce sleep-disturbances, nightmares, flashbacks and hypervigilance, amongst other symptoms, seems overly optimistic, given the pervasive and vicious nature of the injury.) However, many of the study's veteran participants did report positive results in other areas of their lives, particularly self-esteem, self-awareness and improved relationships with others.[97] These findings concur with much of the research on the human-nature relationship presented earlier in this chapter. And the researchers recommended that Outward Bound experiences continue to be made available to veterans.

In 2013, Nevin Harper, Julian Norris and Mark DasTous completed a longitudinal study of Outward Bound Canada's veterans' program, which corroborates the results of previous studies, in terms of the sense of community/camaraderie that develops, the increased self-confidence and the safety and commonality that veterans find through spending time with other veterans. Participants, especially those who described a readiness for change in their lives, continued to experience the benefits of a course six weeks later. The researchers report that "courses have consistently been gateway experiences for participants who subsequently go on to seek out new wellness strategies—ranging from finding peer support to entering an OSI clinic."[98]

In 2013, Israeli researchers also published a study that examined a year-long Nature Adventure Rehabilitation (NAR) program as a supplemental approach to treating war veterans with chronic combat-related post-traumatic stress. Similar to Outward Bound, "NAR happens in a natural environment where participants are faced with a variety of pre-planned tasks and strategies for affecting change."[99] Such approaches typically focus on participants' health rather than their illness. In the Israeli study, groups of six to ten male veterans went on a weekly three-hour sailing trip over a 12-month period. At the end of a year, the results were encouraging. Compared to a control group, the researchers found "medium improvements in [post-traumatic stress], depression, social and emotional quality of life, and large improvements in daily functioning, hope, and [perceived control over illness]." Many veterans in the study also "reported less distress, more moments of 'grace' when they were not bothered by memories or feeling numb, as well as seemed to smile and laugh more often." In addition, an important sense of community developed as the veterans began to connect with and support one another outside their weekly sailing time. Many described, too, how the "sea had a calming effect" and admitted that it became a safe place for them.[100]

In 2009, Jacqueline Atkinson, a professor of public health at the University of Glasgow, conducted an evaluation of the Gardening Leave project, a horticultural therapy program for British Armed Forces veterans. At the time, Gardening Leave was only a pilot project working in association with Hollybush House, a treatment center for veterans in Ayrshire, Scotland. Gardening was considered an adjunct therapy to Hollybush House's regular clinical and non-clinical therapies. Some of the veterans involved said that the project was literally a "life-saver," and reported that they were coping better with their injuries, learning new skills and developing a sense of safety.[101] The Gardening Leave project has since expanded its operations, and today supports veterans' gardens in Erkine and Chelsea, too, with an additional outreach project in East Acton, London.

In 2012, the Danish Centre for Forest, Landscape and Planning at the University of Copenhagen, in partnership with the Stress Center Kalmia, opened The Healing Forest Garden Nacadia (called Nacadia, for short) north of Copenhagen to experiment with taking psychotherapy outdoors. Nacadia features a 3.7-acre healing garden.[102] For researchers, this facility provides an ability to examine the long-term effects of nature-based therapies. University of Copenhagen PhD student Dorthe Varning Poulsen is currently completing a longitudinal study with eight veterans suffering from post-traumatic stress, who took part in a 10-week intervention in Nacadia. Activities, which vary according to season, include working in the garden three times a week, performing mindfulness exercises outdoors, walking in the forest, planting and picking wild berries.[103]

Another new project targeting both Danish and Scottish veterans is Nature Retreat for Veterans, a two-and-a-half-year pilot program established by journalist Anne-Line Ussing and her husband Stuart Press, a retired Australian Army Officer and veteran. In 2001, while working as a UN diplomat, the traumas of deployments to Somalia and particularly Rwanda caught up with Press. He left the UN and bought an organic farm on the island of Strynoe in southern Denmark with his wife. Press soon began to realize the positive effects of farming on his injuries,[104] and the couple is now working to extend those benefits to other veterans. In 2012, Ussing ran a small pilot project on the Falkland Estate in Fife, Scotland, to introduce veterans to conservation work. One participant commented, "It's been good getting away from the flat, getting outdoors, and break the bad habit of sitting indoors. It has been a retreat for me—hanging out with people who are like myself and doing meaningful, practical work."[105] With the two-and-a-half-year pilot program, Ussing and Press will offer introductory courses for veterans on their farm in Denmark, after which veterans will be invited to join veteran-led nature preservation missions in Scotland, Denmark and beyond. The project's intent is to support veterans in realizing safety in nature, to find camaraderie with other veterans, to engage veterans in meaningful activities and to provide new skills that improve veterans' employment opportunities.

⊕ ⊕ ⊕

The veterans' stories shared in the next chapters give space to former soldiers' personal experiences and realizations that their interconnections with nature provide alternative experiences to their military training and combat exposure. The importance of paying attention to these stories is that, as outlined above, they corroborate similar experiences of a growing number of veterans and point toward an avenue of recovery that is little acknowledged in conventional therapeutic and medical interventions. Overall, veterans' nature-based activities have shown them the way forward—the ways that life can continue beyond their military experiences—and as Andy Fisher told me, these narratives lead us to think about what else "might be called for in the healing process."

Getting Back to Our Roots

Nathan Lewis and the Veterans' Sanctuary

Nathan Lewis is one of the founders of the Veterans' Sanctuary, a project that includes a garden, a writing group and a paper-making initiative, all to support veterans from the wars in Iraq and Afghanistan as they transition to civilian life. The veterans' main goal for the garden is sustainable food security: to grow high-quality food for themselves, and to share with their friends, allies in the community and other veterans. "There are not many fixes, and gardening's not a fix, but it's an effort," said Nathan. "It gives you a fighting chance. It keeps you in the game. It allows you to take control of your own situation, of your own destiny."[1]

❀ ❀ ❀

"It's really nice at the end of the day to stop and look at what your labor has produced," said Iraq war veteran Nathan Lewis. "To look at something tangible and, without a doubt, positive. Because, in the military, I don't feel like I served my country in Iraq. I feel like I served Big Oil. I think, for myself and a lot of other veterans, we are just looking for meaningful ways to serve." It was a Monday evening in early November 2012, and Nathan had just spent the day working at the Veterans' Sanctuary community garden in Trumansburg, outside of Ithaca, New York. The Veterans' Sanctuary garden was at one time only a dream shared by Nathan and several other veterans. They imagined creating a positive space for veterans to come together, to plan, share, work and communicate and to combat the loneliness and isolation that plagues many veterans upon returning home from war and reintegrating into civilian life. Now in its fourth season, that positive space has become a reality.

Nathan, who suffers from service-related post-traumatic stress, summarized the main benefits of working in the garden: "A lot of vets have trouble sleeping, and I have here and there, but if I'm outside with a shovel for 8 to 10 hours, and especially doing it as a labor of love," Nathan explained, "I don't have trouble sleeping anymore. I want to be out there, so I have no problem whatsoever cranking out a 10- or 12-hour day, and then sleep comes real easy." He laughed. "It's just real basic stuff—moving your body and eating good food. Often it's the most overlooked. I go to the VA and they want to give me pills for everything. And I smile and say, 'No thank you, I'm good.' Not everyone can do that, but I can."

As its name implies, the Veterans' Sanctuary garden is a place that Nathan finds incredibly peaceful, but perhaps more importantly, it's a place he feels safe. A sense of safety is lacking for many veterans suffering from post-traumatic stress, and it's something most savor when they find it. In addition to working the soil and tending the plants, all the other projects that come with keeping up a large garden and two greenhouses provide "a lot of anchors into life," Nathan told me. "If you're feeling bad, and you're feeling shitty and you're suicidal, you feel very alone and gloomy, anything that keeps you strapped into this world—into the living—is good. I can't go nowhere because the beets need watering and the chickens need to be fed. And that's all I can think to do. I've seen too many people go off, fall apart, kill themselves or just drop out of life—and it's sad," Nathan told me. "I'm not a trained psychologist, but I do know that just starting with this real simple basic stuff, like good nutrition and collaborative projects and trying to recreate the village that has been destroyed, [is helpful]."

Whenever Nathan needs a boost in his spirits, or feels the need to recharge, he heads out to the garden. "I just go out there alone and shovel in the wheelbarrow for a few hours and feel great about a lot of things—feel great about life. It doesn't need to be more complicated than that; it's just a grounding thing, getting back to our roots," he commented. "Everyone's got farmers in their family. Everyone. And I think Gandhi had a lot of wisdom saying something about everyone should have a hand in the food production because they'll respect it more, have a stronger connection to the Earth and be grounded. You really quickly understand how much work goes into garlic and how much to respect it, and know how useful it is. You totally look at food in a different way when you start growing your own."

There was no sudden epiphany for Nathan that gardening was improving his health and his overall outlook on life while also reducing his post-traumatic stress symptoms. "It was just slow and steady," he observed. However, he does recall being introduced to a European-style scythe the first year he and his friends started the Veterans' Sanctuary garden. "I ordered it and used it that first summer, mowing with the scythe and then raking all the cuttings into a bed—a really, really large square bed where we eventually planted garlic—that, to me, was the coolest thing ever! We didn't have to plow it, we didn't have to use shovels to turn the soil; we just kept layering freshly cut grass and putting straw and manure on it, and then eventually it was this really fertile bed where we grew garlic. I think that was an 'aha' moment that yes, this feels good, this feels right. And just going there and doing it and trying it every day. It's rewarding."

🍃 🍃 🍃

Nathan grew up in a family of five children in Barker, Niagara County, in western New York State. During his high-school years, army recruiters came to his school regularly, where, he told me, they continue to do very well. "Not many jobs, careers, cultural opportunities for people in areas like that," he said. And so, in 2001 right out of high school—and like many of his peers—Nathan enlisted in the US Army field artillery for two years. As he described it now, "I was coaxed into joining the military; it wasn't something I really sought out. It wasn't my own idea." He left for basic training in Fort Sill, Oklahoma, in August 2001. Then September 11 happened. Nathan recalled training hard in the year leading up to the Iraq War, and he was deployed in March 2003. After a brief time in Kuwait, his unit went to Baghdad, where they spent the next five months collecting weapons and ammunitions stockpiles in the immediate aftermath of the invasion. "We were trying to police up all the weapons stockpiles so they wouldn't fall into the hands of the insurgents," said Nathan. "So we spent a lot of time on the roads, a lot of time going into bunkers, buildings and Iraqi army bases, into warehouses and in the streets, just handling weapons and explosives and putting them on the trucks and kicking them off somewhere safer."

Nathan had strong reservations about the war from the start, and once in Iraq, he wanted to get out as soon as possible. In August 2003, his two-year enlistment period was up. "All I had to do to get out was not reenlist." However, he remembers the period immediately following his return home as an "unsteady, dark, troubling time." He was very unhappy and suffered from extreme anger. The next few years were filled with heavy drinking, substance abuse and bar fights. Nathan also experienced deep guilt about his participation in the war. "As the war unfolded and as the violence increased, as different scandals came to light, whether they be massacres of unarmed civilians, or torture in the prisons, or the Battle of Fallujah, I started to really, really get a gut-wrenching guilt, and I was just sick of the whole thing."

After leaving the Army, Nathan began attending the local community college, but he felt alienated from his civilian peers who did not share his experiences. "They didn't seem to know anything about it or care. They didn't seem to know the war was still going on, and would often ask inappropriate questions if anything at all." He also held several jobs, including one at the local lumber yard, but felt alienated from his co-workers there, too, who upon learning he was a veteran, often expressed what Nathan called "racist and genocidal" opinions about killing everyone in the Middle East or turning the entire region into a parking lot.

Through his struggles, Nathan eventually found his way to the group Iraq Veterans Against the War (IVAW), in which he was active between 2006 and 2008. In contrast to the alienation he felt around his college peers and lumber yard co-workers, Nathan felt at home amongst IVAW veterans who shared his experiences and whom he described as "progressively minded, interesting people, looking to do different things and not afraid to rock the boat."

Nathan and a small group of others often discussed their desire to settle down together on a farm and to create a peer-to-peer program to support veterans reintegrating into civilian life. While they imagined different possibilities and programs, growing their own food was always central to the conversation. And Nathan was no stranger to gardening. When he was growing up, his family had a large garden in which they grew mostly annuals and some fruit trees, and he, along with his twin brother and three sisters, spent plenty of time weeding and hoeing in the garden. The family also had a small but popular roadside stand where they sold Lewis Sweet Corn.

By the time he had completed community college, Nathan continued to harbor a deep distrust in the economy and many of the traditional, popular cultural assumptions and beliefs held in US society. "I felt very unstable and insecure in terms of the basics in life—food, shelter and money. I was looking to do something different, so subsistence farming really spoke to me." And based on past experiences, he was not eager to find another job. "I just felt like dropping out of society and the economy," he explained. "And so I was really primed to start working at the Sanctuary."

Along with a few friends, Nathan put together what would eventually become the Veterans' Sanctuary, a 501(c)(3) non-profit. They chose Ithaca, New York, as their base because of their connections in the community within the anti-war movement, and also its reputation as a progressive, radical community supportive of veterans' issues. Initially, the friends hoped to buy some land, but they lacked the finances. Eager to get started, they kept themselves open to alternative possibilities, and fortune was on their side. "We figured out that capital wasn't necessarily a critical element in putting something like this together," Nathan recalled. "We just got lucky and met the right person who knew of some land that had two enormous greenhouses on it."

The two- to three-acre parcel in Trumansburg, just outside of Ithaca, had not been used for some time. Trees grew up through the greenhouse floors, weeds and trash were everywhere, and soil fertility was generally poor. But it was enough to get started. Nathan, his friends and the landowner made an agreement on a handshake, and the Veterans' Sanctuary

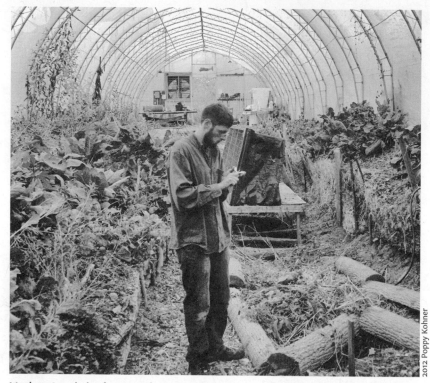

2012 Poppy Kohner

Nathan Lewis in the greenhouse at the Veterans' Sanctuary

garden was born. The veterans were to act as caretakers of the land and to leave it in better condition than when they started. Nathan described the seven-year lease agreement with the landowners as "a very healthy collaboration, cooperative effort. They're not trying to squeeze rent out of us. They donate the land. Once in a while, we take them a basket of vegetables or fruit or whatever's around, but pretty much we just have access to it."

That first year, the veterans cleaned up the land. They built raised beds and planted a variety of food crops, with a particular focus on long-term fruit and berries and cold-hearty perennials, which tend to be more disease- and drought-resistant than annuals. These included reliable crops such as horseradish, nettles and Jerusalem artichokes. Reflecting on growing Jerusalem artichokes, Nathan laughed: "I don't even necessarily like them all that much. I've found a few ways to cook them and ferment them, but they always give you gas and they don't taste the best. But there's just something really awesome about going out with a shovel, cracking open the soil in whatever month that you want to, throwing them in there and then they come up. And then you try to dig them up, and they're doubled the next year. It's like the Terminator, they just keep coming back; you just can't mess with them!"

The veterans' main goal for their garden is sustainable food security. "We like to think about and follow a lot of permaculture principles to try to integrate things, instead of just big monocrops. We don't have any power tools except a chainsaw," Nathan explained. "I like not having a tractor. I like not smelling fumes. Talk about triggers and shit—diesel exhaust makes me think of the fuckin' Army, that's universal! That's kind of the hallmark of the military, that you smell diesel exhaust. So we really value the marginal things. The whole space is kind of a marginal space; if you were starting a for-profit farm, you wouldn't look at the place where we farm now. We want to be independent and fairly resilient. So we try to get stuff, and saving seeds is just one of the many things we're trying to learn and get good at."

In an ideal world, Nathan said, the Veterans' Sanctuary would include animals in their operation. "If I had a whole homestead somewhere, without a doubt I'd get some goats or some sheep or chickens and ducks," he told me. And several years ago, the group did experiment with incorporating laying hens into the garden. The chickens lived in the greenhouse for a time, and then in chicken tractors (which are chicken coops without a floor that can be moved around to different areas). However, because none of the veterans live at the garden space, they are limited in their ability to care for animals, and after about a year, they realized that keeping chickens was not practical. "We were going through a pretty chaotic time where we weren't able to take care of them that well, so we ate them."

To learn the different skills associated with farming and permaculture, the veterans take an experiential approach—talking to other farmers, reading books—and trial and error. Sometimes they succeed, and other times they fail. Nathan pointed to the group's latest experiments implementing a humanure system.

"What's that?" I asked. "I'm not familiar with that term."

"Humanure…" Nathan hesitated briefly, and the awareness of what he was talking about suddenly dawned on me. "You're basically composting your human waste. It's intentional in the sense that you're going to be using that as fertilizer. I just think it's awesome; not everyone does." Nathan went on to describe the reactions of friends to the veterans' latest experiment. "Usually it's at dinner when we start bragging: 'Yeah we're shittin' in buckets, and we're gonna have some awesome fertilizer.' And their chewing slows down, and they kind of look at you. But then I look at them and say, 'Oh no, you have to wait a year, just to be safe, so we haven't fertilized anything yet.' So they're like, 'Oh, good, this food isn't fertilized with shit.' 'No, it's not.' 'Oh, OK, good, good, good.' So there are still a lot of taboos with that sort of thing."

By the end of the year, they had collected two large compost bins of humanure. "We made really nice containers for it; it was really neat and orderly. And they did get hot, they were certainly cooking down," Nathan explained. But when the veterans moved out of their shared house in January 2013, they couldn't take the compost because it was winter, and they worried that the new renters would want to keep it. "So we went back to the old house with a plan that we were going to say, 'Hey, we left our compost here. Do you mind if we haul it out? And if they said, 'Yeah,' then good, we wouldn't mention that it was humanure," said Nathan. "But if they said, 'No, we want to use it,' we were going to pull that out of our back pockets and say, 'Well actually it's not compost, but we were crapping in buckets for a year,'" he laughed heartily. "Luckily it didn't come down to that. All we had to do was pick it up."

They moved the humanure compost out to the farm, and mixed it with grass cuttings. Nathan explained that they are continuing to collect and compost it, but haven't used the initial batch yet because it was not completely composted. "It's still cooking down, and we have full intention to incorporate that right into the farm—especially by next spring, it will be broken down enough where you won't be able to tell what it was. Not that you could tell when we were shovelling it; it looked like any other half-finished compost," Nathan said. "So it's moving in a good direction. We'll get to it someday."

⊕ ⊕ ⊕

Given that their main goal is sustainable food security, the veterans are particularly focused on growing food for the members of the Veterans' Sanctuary and then sharing what's left over with their friends, allies in the community and other veterans. "We share with the local food bank when we can. We give it to veterans and their families in town when we can. Just today we gave some to an outreach coordinator from the Binghamton Vet Center. They have a nutrition and cooking class with veterans down at the Vet Center in Binghamton, and so it felt really good to give them a bunch of kale and daikon radishes and onions because they're going to learn to cook and prepare it, and say, 'Hey, these vets have this farm up there and they grew this!'" However, the importance of growing their own food runs deeper than food security, Nathan told me. "It's not only food security but to have real food that is healing and nourishes bodies, so veterans can get their nutrients and have a fighting chance to tackle some of the more long-term, deeper spiritual/soul/war trauma issues, to try to sort them out. I see it as very important: first things first—your body has to be nourished. You have to exercise."

Since starting the garden, the members of Veterans' Sanctuary have come a long way. They are now eating a lot of the food they grow. "I'm starting to benefit a lot in terms of health and payoffs, which provides the motivation to keep me doing it." They started with small, limited goals and have been expanding very slowly. "We try to move forward with a very low footprint, so we're not trying to build large outbuildings or anything like that. We try to generally just improve the land, so that means mowing, and if a tree comes down, we're the ones that clean it up. Once in a while, we ask the landowners' permission to do something, but mostly we have a whole lot of autonomy and trust. We just do what we feel is best, and it works out."

Their practices as a group have also evolved. In the beginning, two or three veterans would go to the garden whenever they had time. Today, the Veterans' Sanctuary advertises and invites anyone in the community to come out to the garden to work with them on Mondays. While their outreach efforts are focused primarily toward veterans living in the Ithaca area, the group of Monday gardeners is usually mixed, with both veterans and non-veterans, and can vary in size from 2 to 15 people.

The veterans who come out are usually a demographically mixed group. "There are Vietnam vets all the way to the present conflict. There are female vets, combat, non-combat, deployed, non-deployed, all different branches." In addition, every few weeks, veterans from other parts of the country pass through the area, stop and stay a while to work in the garden. Overall though, Nathan told me, "We're still a small group. We need help very badly. It's hard to get people that have enough open time to do all the work with the farm."

The need for help became especially real during the 2013 growing season. After moving out of their collective rental house in January, where ½ to ¾ of the tenants had been in the military at some time, the veterans no longer benefited from low rent that allowed them to spend plenty of time in the garden. "Obviously that's a huge problem for people, myself included: the ability to have to work to make ends meet and cover the basics in life. Unless you have a really good financial situation without having to do 40- or 50-hour workweeks, it's really difficult to be able to give a day or half a day a week to some kind of community project," said Nathan, who in 2013 cut back on the amount of time he spent in the garden because he found steady work at a tree service, alongside other odd jobs in the community. Reflecting on his current situation, he told me, "It's good because I have a little more stability, but it's at the expense of spending more hours at the farm." Also, since many of his friends work on farms, he explained, "the last thing they want after pulling garlic all day is to come out to the Veterans' Sanctuary garden and pull more garlic.

"But we still have a core group of 4 or 5, maybe 10 people who come sporadically but consistently, so we still have enough to keep going. We're just really trying to expand the organizing crew, to put that responsibility on more than one or two people," Nathan explained. "We've had to prioritize and really focus on a few things that we consider very important. Garlic and potatoes are the two things this year that we've been focusing on. So we've been doing good, just rolling with it and not getting too discouraged."

Adding to their difficulties, groundhogs ate this year's plantings of lettuce and kale. Nathan suspects that the groundhogs are doing so well because of the increased food supply, both from the gardens and the compost donated by the community. "And some people in our group have an aversion to killing them—myself included. I used a crossbow to kill two, but it was not a very fun experience, so I don't find myself finding a whole lot of time to do that." Still, Nathan said, "we're rolling with it," and told how they are learning to identify and appreciate wild, edible weeds, such as dandelions, sorrel, purslane and pokeweed shoots. "We've also planted more things that the groundhogs don't like—horse-radish and perennial onions—and things like that."

⊕ ⊕ ⊕

Every Sunday while they were living together, the veterans hosted a pot-luck for Veterans' Sanctuary members and friends. "It's cool to share a lot of the food that we grow, that our friends help us grow, with our general circle of friends, our general community," Nathan explained. Before sitting down to eat together, they reviewed the contents of the meal to show what their labor had produced. Generally, very little of the food was bought from the grocery store; most often, between 70 and 100% was grown in their garden or traded for, or their friends grew or traded for, or someone gave them.

Indeed, non-cash transactions, labor trades and other possibilities outside the current economic system have been essential to the Veterans' Sanctuary. Nathan reiterated his own sense of distrust in the current system. "I just distrust a lot of the ways people do things," he remarked. "Also, I just can't afford good food." He mused that if he did not grow his own food, buying the high-quality organic food that he eats now would take up much of his budget. "So why not just avoid that whole hassle? Just work directly to get the food, or the shelter, the necessities of life, not going through lots of people in the middle."

While the greenhouse helps to extend their growing season in up-state New York, over the winter months, the members of the Veterans' Sanctuary concentrate primarily on the other aspects of their program. "The winter is my time to write and make paper," explained Nathan. Twice a month, the Veterans' Sanctuary organizes for local veterans to come together to write, and when we last spoke, they were preparing to publish a book of poetry. In addition, they make handmade "combat pa-per" out of their army uniforms and work clothes. Nathan spent much of January and February 2013 making paper, and he expected that most of the following winter would be spent printing his book—a small edi-tion of 250 books, each with 10 individual prints using a variety of print-ing techniques. As the Veterans' Sanctuary programs develop, there is also some overlap between the different projects. For example, Nathan hopes to eventually plant a dye garden and grow plants that can be used to make paper. "We're trying to keep an eye on everything, and we try to think about sustainability and go low-impact as much as possible on all our different projects."

The most difficult part of the Veterans' Sanctuary's community gar-den project is that, while it's a lot of work, it doesn't pay. "You can grow your own food, and if you're trying to do like we are—to subsist as much as you can off of it—it's really hard to come up with money for rent and other stuff because so much of your time is spent on the farm. So the financial realities are pretty tough to overcome." At the same time, gar-dening doesn't require a lot of capital, and almost anyone can grow a garden. "You just stop mowing a part of your lawn and put something in there." But Nathan also raised the point that many communities in North America have laws against people growing food in their front yard. "What's this food doing here? Get it out of here!" he chuckled, mimicking a bylaw officer. "It's hard for people to break out of their norms."

When I ask about the benefits of small-scale organic farming for vet-erans beyond those involved in the Veterans' Sanctuary, Nathan sug-gested that it's part of a larger movement to change the North American food system. "The alternative would be big agribusiness, which is a terri-bly stressful, destructive thing. On a not-for-profit farm, we can avoid all the hassles, the headaches and the stress. And just enjoy the work, enjoy the food and get the most out of it." Moreover many veterans, according to Nathan, are looking for ways to make sense of their lives and experi-ences. "I think there are a lot of people that want to nurture instead of destroy with their hands. So obviously the organic methods speak to that and fulfill that wish far more than the other way," he observed.

Most importantly, Nathan continued to emphasize the importance of good nutrition. It is important for everyone, he believes, but perhaps even more so for veterans and their families. "Especially for veterans that have high levels of stress, exposure to environmental toxins. Their families are under more stress because of deployment, and it's absolutely necessary that they get good food. And what's even better is that they have a hand in that food, have that relationship with the dirt and know where things come from. And it's a great way to build a community, whether it's a single vet or a vet with a family. If you have a family, it's a way that you can work together on something that is very, very rewarding. It's a lasting, tangible accomplishment—and the interest on it starts to compound and really build up."

On the topic of veterans' exposure to environmental toxins, Nathan became suddenly angry as he shared the story of his friend, also an Iraq War veteran, who recently died of cancer at age 32. The doctors attributed the cancer to his exposure to burn pits, which were used at military bases in both Iraq and Afghanistan to burn garbage, including various chemicals, plastics, oils, metals, paper and other waste, thus releasing contaminants into the air surrounding the base. "You can't find a vet that wasn't around the fuckin' burn pits. It's bullshit!" Nathan exclaimed. "I feel like an Agent Orange-type epidemic is coming, or it's already here, so I think of food as absolutely necessary. I feel like I don't have a choice besides eating super high-quality food, working outside almost year-round and staying physically very active and healthy...figuring out the stuff that might fix what was put in."

In addition, for Nathan, farming and gardening offer effective and worthwhile opportunities for veterans' healing and reintegration into society. Working with the soil and cultivating good food provide meaningful work, which is difficult for many veterans to find in current economic times. Nathan emphasized his desire to see gardens and farms run by the VA—or other organizations—across the US. "I guarantee that there are probably thousands of vets who would be happy to put down the pills and start figuring out herbal remedies. And be involved in learning about them and drying them and using them and showing other people them. I think people need to be empowered to say, 'This is my health. The VA ain't gonna fix me.' If you're feeling like shit, you need to talk to someone, or you need to figure out some real deep soul-searching—to love yourself again—the VA isn't going to give you that. You have to figure it out for yourself!"

Nathan also believes there is a lot to be learned from working with the soil and plants, and the ways that the Earth slowly heals and regenerates itself through composting. "The Earth has things built in that no matter what we do, it can slowly heal itself and fix itself," he said, suggesting that the Earth provides a model for veterans' own healing and recovery. In addition, Nathan told me, the community experience of working in the garden is important. "I don't know if I'd do it if it was just me out there. It's too overwhelming, but with a group effort, that's a really cool thing. You've gotta plan things out. You've gotta talk. You've gotta communicate. You've gotta work together, all those things. We're social creatures."

Nathan then reiterated the importance of using hand tools in the garden for his own recovery, the ways that hand tools keep him anchored into life. "Using a tool, even a simple hoe or shovel, is therapy. It makes you happy. It's on a very basic level, like eating and shitting, it's all part of it, that's what I love about it. People don't even realize it. Some of my friends that come out—the vets—sometimes they're not so into it [at first]. They'll make all these comments and act like it's the most terrible thing ever and ask 'why are we doing this?' But then you catch them smiling and laughing, and they come back. It's just like a kid that eats something and they didn't think they liked it, and then they eat it and they say, 'This is pretty good.' See? I told ya!" Nathan laughed again.

Gardening is a proactive activity that has enabled Nathan to take responsibility for his own healing and recovery. "The tools are in your hands. Look no further than the ends of your arms. It's empowering; it puts the ball in your court. It's not some pills. It's not a counselor who's going to tell you things that'll fix you; it just doesn't work like that. People need to build up their self-esteem. They need to be excited about things. They need a dream. They need to be exhausted and sleep! They don't need pills that make them into zombies so they can't dream and they can't sleep, they can't get excited, they can't connect with people because it turns them into these monsters, and all the stigma that goes with that, too. Always taking pills, always hearing that you're a disorder—they call it a *disorder*, post-traumatic stress disorder. There's no disorder in the condition. It's your natural body and soul's reaction to a very brutal and unjust war." Referring to the Iraq War, Nathan declared, "It's unbelievable what happened over there, what people come home with and what they have to live with. There are not many fixes, and gardening's not a fix but it's an effort. It gives you a fighting chance. It keeps you in the game. It allows you to take control of your own situation, of your own destiny. Otherwise it's always 'someone else': someone else sent you over there, someone else told you what to do, someone else told you to shoot somebody, and someone else gave you a pill to fix it all, and someone else is telling you that it's a disorder and you're broken."

While like many veterans, Nathan is critical of the VA, and particularly its strong emphasis on medication as the fix for veterans' health issues, Nathan does acknowledge that it has a place. "We do benefit in a lot of ways. They do what they can, and it's full of really well-intentioned people." Still, he hopes that the Veterans' Sanctuary will come to serve as another kind of health care model for veterans and others who are suffering. "People can look at us and say, 'Holy shit, they have almost no budget a year.' If our yearly budget for the garden is $1,500, that's a huge budget to us! And to do the amount of stuff we do on the resources we have, I think it's pretty amazing. But it would be even better if the VAs and different institutions would support it and help it along. I'd love a salary for what I do. It would be awesome. I'd be there a lot more." Indeed, it is Nathan's hope that someday soon, "every VA will have a farm somewhere close, and there'll be dozens and dozens of vets on any given sunny day out there farming."

Nathan's definitive advice to other veterans? "Don't be afraid of trying something new." But he recommended starting slowly, avoiding the urge to take on too much at first. "As with anything important in life, if you don't keep committed to it and working at it, it will usually entropy and devolve and fall apart," he said. In hindsight, he wishes that the Veterans' Sanctuary had spent more time developing systems that could maintain themselves during times when the veterans needed more focus in other areas of their lives. "There's this initial euphoria of 'Oh, this is going to be awesome.' Everyone's got ideas, and you try to do them all and next thing you know, there are half dug holes everywhere and 20 different kinds of onions." Nathan laughed. At the same time, he acknowledged that, as an experiential learner, intense planning is not his style. "I'd rather do some prior reading and research and a whole lot of hands-on doing. It's not the most efficient way, but it's certainly the most exciting!"

4

Peace by the River

Christian McEachern and the
Canadian Veteran Adventure Foundation

*Christian McEachern served as a peacekeeper in the former Yugoslavia and
Uganda, and was diagnosed with PTSD in 1997. After hitting rock bottom in
2001, he has spent the last 13 years rebuilding his life. It was in 2005 as Christian sat on the banks of the Columbia River that he finally felt "at peace with
life for a moment," and he realized that outdoor experiences were something
missing from veterans' care. In response, he founded the Canadian Veteran
Adventure Foundation (CVAF), which he envisioned would provide another
tier in veterans' care through outdoor programming and adventure training.
Christian also recognizes the profound importance of both dogs and horses
in his own journey toward recovery.[1]*

The first time I interviewed Cpl (Ret.) Christian McEachern, C.D., it
was one of those warm January days that occasionally bless us on the
east side of the Rocky Mountains. As I drove southwest of Calgary to
meet Christian at the house he was renting near Priddis with a friend,
I was awed by the stunning beauty in this part of the world: brilliant
sun and cloudless winter blue sky against the crisp white snow-covered
mountains. Christian met me by the barn at the top of the hill where I
parked my car. I was eight months pregnant, and he didn't want me to
fall on the icy pathway leading down to the house; he also made sure
I wasn't bowled over by his two large dogs, Nevada and Buddy, who
rushed to greet me.

After a few minutes of casual conversation, we settled into his living room, with its wall of windows overlooking the foothills and the mountains. "I was a good soldier. I was doing everything everybody else was," Christian told me. In his early 40s, unshaven with greying hair, fit and wearing casual outdoor clothing, Christian presented an image similar to many of the avid "outdoorsy-types" who live in and around Calgary. If I passed him in the street, it would not occur to me that he was a veteran, or that he suffers from occupational stress injury (OSI). Although soft-spoken, his frustration was clear. "For the most part, I was outstanding with the top marks you could get as a soldier, but after a couple of tours, I was partying hard like everybody else and started losing focus."

When he was young, Christian imagined he would grow up to be a paramedic. But after starting Cadets at age 12, he knew he wanted to be in the military. At 17, he joined the Reserves, followed by the regular Canadian Forces, where he spent the next 14 years serving as a member of the Princess Patricia's Canadian Light Infantry (PPCLI), including UN-sanctioned peacekeeping missions in the former Yugoslavia and Uganda. On both missions, Christian witnessed or was subject to a number of horrifying events, leading to his PTSD diagnosis in 1997. He was animated and candid as he spoke about his experiences as a young soldier in training and on peacekeeping missions.

"When I did my leadership course in 1993 before I deployed to Yugoslavia, it was 3 months of high stress. We started with almost 60 people and graduated with 12, and most of them were medical or physical failures. It was 24-hours-a-day, 5-days-a-week of sleep deprivation. You'd go home, sleep Friday night, live fire all day Saturday," he recalled. "Sunday was a recoup day, although it was cleaning gear and getting yelled at and lockers being thrown around and shit like that, but after three months I came home and my girlfriend at the time was like, 'You're a fuckin' mess!'"

At home, Christian would sometimes find himself shaking his then-girlfriend awake. "I'd be trying to wake her up for her shift, saying, 'Come on, get up, it's your fucking shift.' There were just strange things, where she'd find me crawling around on the floor trying to find my rifle, because if it's anywhere farther away from you than grabbing distance, you're in serious trouble. They train you so hard that it's instinct after a while," he said, "and this isn't even combat, this is just what they're training guys to do, and it starts to affect your home life."

After completing leadership training, Christian was part of a peace-keeping tour in the former Yugoslavia. "You're working 22 or 23 hours a day on the front line, being shot at or guys are getting killed or wounded with land mines," he recollected, then added, "So, by the time I came home after about a year and a half in Yugoslavia and with all the leadership training, I was pretty wired. And the thing was it wasn't just me, it was everybody. They trained us hard for Yugoslavia as if we were going to war, and then we came home from Yugoslavia and were pretty disgusted with the blue beret, the United Nations and the rules of engagement. Not that we wanted to go over and shoot people, but we did want to go over and make a difference."

Christian had no opportunity to spend money on the front lines, other than a weekend break in Budapest and a week in Holland, and Christian remembers coming home from Yugoslavia at age 24 with $35,000 in his bank account. "For the most part, you come home, you're young, you're completely wired, you're feeling invincible," he said. "It wasn't that we were bad people or that we wanted to hurt anybody, but when you do the sleep deprivation stuff…I've driven vehicles so tired that drunk driving is easy. The guys just start to push themselves. I don't have any trouble talking about this; I'm ashamed of some of the stuff that I did, but you have to realize that it was also a lot of the environment that we were in."

Shortly after coming home from Yugoslavia, Christian and his army buddies were partying hard and beginning to get into bar fights. "It wasn't that I was starting them, or some of my buddies were starting them, but when you get these civvies pushing you and pushing you and pushing you, and you get an army guy who's that close to being wired already—and so we finished a few fights pretty good." And at that point, Christian said, "the assault charges started coming in—assault causing bodily harm and all this kind of stuff—and at the time I didn't think too much of it. In fact, nobody thought anything of it, that a lot of guys

were getting violent charges and stuff against them. I don't know anything about what was going on in home lives with families, obviously,
because I wasn't a family guy, but as a single guy, I was seven-days-a-
week partying. You could still do your job, but you were making more
self-destructive decisions," he told me. "When you look back at my dos-
sier at when I got in trouble at particular times, it was all related to either
right after an operation or after a significant event within the military."

In 1997, Christian decided to see a military doctor, but only because
he thought he might be having a heart attack. It turned out he was having panic attacks. "I'd be training guys out in the bush, and I'd come back
off a night patrol at four o'clock in the morning, and usually I'd get about
an hour's sleep before first light, which kicks everything awake again,
and I'd be rolling over having nightmares, and my recruits would look
over and I'd be drenched in sweat, sitting on my pack, with my rifle up,
and the guys were like, 'Are you OK?' You have to shake your head and
go, 'OK, right, I'm in Canada.' It starts to blend together," Christian said.
"It took a few years, but when you look back at the progression of it,
there were definitely a lot of signs that I wasn't right in the head when I
got home."

Christian was honorably discharged from the Canadian Forces in
2001. He knows that his post-traumatic struggles will be part of his life's
journey for a long time, and he provided insight into what life is like
for him now. "Sometimes I just get really tired," he admitted. "I'm not
good with the emotional rollercoaster stuff, the highs and the lows." He
disclosed that, like many others suffering from post-traumatic stress, he
does not sleep well, often getting only a few hours of sleep each night
for months at a time. And then there are the "nightmares, which happen nightly, they never go away, I wish they would." After hitting rock
bottom in 2001, Christian has been coping better over the years, but admitted that he's still "not out of the woods." He still feels isolated, often
prefers spending time with animals over people, and all in all, confessed
that the years since leaving the military have been lonely: "You start to
feel pretty alone on the journey."

And like many veterans, Christian found himself disillusioned with
the civilian world. "I felt like I got better for a while, and then I lost faith

in people again." He looks forward to one day being his own boss. "The army trains us to be really strong leaders. We've got ethics and morals about how people should be treated, and I haven't seen a lot of it on the outside world. It seems like everyone is trying to take advantage of everybody else."

🍃 🍃 🍃

A few years after leaving the Canadian Forces, Christian began studying for a Bachelor of Applied Ecotourism and Outdoor Leadership (ETOL) at Mount Royal College (now Mount Royal University) in Calgary, Alberta. Ian Sherrington, an associate professor in the ETOL program, remembered having Christian in his classes. "He was a phenomenal student from the beginning," said Ian. "Obviously very different from the other students, with an incredibly different perspective. He was much older—at least 10, 12, 14 years older than all the other students—and also had this myriad of life experiences that the other students didn't have…that most people in the world don't have. So I think he struggled in some ways, and in other ways he tried to fit in."[2]

Christian confessed that he initially felt worried and anxious—common emotions amongst stress-injured veterans—about how he would do in the ETOL program. "I was quite worried about performing for some of the bigger tasks, like climbing a mountain again and having a panic attack," he told me. "When you go from being able to do anything you want to taking a knee in Safeway because you're having panic attacks, it really gives you some severe performance anxiety because you're used to being up at this level," he motioned high with his hand, "and you're crawling on the ground like a baby."

He recalled training hard for the course's first expedition in August 2005. "It was almost like I was going out for a mountain warfare course with the Army, which is pretty hard, and of course, once I got there, I quickly realized that I wasn't out of my element, and that I was starting to fit in a little bit. It was just nice." The group started off on the Columbia River in British Columbia. "It's a big wildlife corridor," said Christian, recalling the many animals they saw on the trip. "And after a couple of days, I thought, 'Wow, this is amazing!' and I'm enjoying the activities with the group, and the activity of being outside. It's sunny, in BC...how can you go wrong?"

After going through the entire veteran side of the military system, including counseling and medication, Christian described how it was as he sat on the banks of the Columbia River that he finally felt "at peace with life for a moment." He said he "realized that this was a gap that could be filled, and maybe it would be helpful for other veterans to be able to sit here on the river bank, too." In fact, as he participated in the program's outdoor expeditions, Ian Sherrington, who was Christian's instructor on that first expedition as well as subsequent ones, told how he saw a change in Christian. "It was almost as if I realized I could still do it," said Christian. "I went from being really quiet, in the background, to starting to become a prominent leader in the program. I was trained out here, so I'm good at it, but the confidence wasn't there. Once the confidence started coming back, that's where I started noticing lots of changes."

In their second year, the ETOL students were required to design their own outdoor program, including detailed marketing plans. Most students just imagined a program for the purpose of the assignments, but Christian began applying his assignments toward planning a real outdoor program for veterans. His professors encouraged his passion, and the basic structure of what would eventually become the Canadian Veteran Adventure Foundation took shape.

Christian, along with his friend Monica Culic, founded the non-profit Canadian Veteran Adventure Foundation (CVAF) in 2006. They envisioned it would provide another tier in the care and treatment of Canadian Forces veterans suffering from post-traumatic stress through outdoor programming and adventure training. While Veterans Affairs Canada currently treats veterans with post-traumatic stress with prescription drugs and personal and group therapy, Christian and Monica's vision was that the CVAF would provide a third course of treatment and support for veterans through outdoor programming. They did not see the CVAF's outdoor programs as a "fix" to all the veterans' problems, but rather as compatible with, and capable of enhancing, the effects of medication and therapy.

Importantly, Christian emphasized that the CVAF did not aim to provide gruelling outdoor experiences to veterans. "Outdoor pursuits don't have to be going and climbing a mountain right away. I'm not going to be taking a guy with panic attacks and hanging him off the side of the mountain and telling him to get over it." It's important to consider both the veterans' physical and emotional fitness levels, and to pay careful attention that programs and expeditions do not exceed these levels. "The guys that I'm dealing with, they're too beat up and too abused, they don't want to be pushed," he explained. "Knowing how hard and how far you can push people is pretty important."

Christian also reflected on the low level of trust amongst veterans suffering from post-traumatic stress. "If you don't have face time with them, they're not going to trust you. If you don't have the opportunity to address their concerns face to face, or explain what's going to happen, they automatically think I'm going to take them out and drag them through a commando course in the mountains, so guys aren't going to show up. And especially if they don't trust you, they don't want to go out there and look stupid, having a panic attack on the river, so that's why a lot of the guys will turn down activities like this, because they're so worried about looking stupider than they already feel." Accordingly, Christian worries about programs run by organizations or people who don't have a good understanding of veterans' post-traumatic experience. "It wouldn't surprise me that somebody gets pushed too hard, too fast, by somebody who doesn't know exactly the parameters." Christian said, "Because of where I've come from, I have a real understanding of what they are going through."

In 2007, the CVAF put a horse-drawn wagon in the Calgary Stampede Parade for the families of veterans serving in Afghanistan. Monica Culic, the CVAF's secretary and communications director, recalled that day. "We got a couple of veterans' families through connections at the OSI [operational stress injury] clinic here in town, and they came out and they were thrilled. It was a beautiful day and hot, and one of the veterans had just come back from Afghanistan. And he said, 'You know, a month ago, I was like: 'I was home, no one knows, no one cares what I've done.' And now I'm walking in the Parade with my family and being treated like I'm important and that really meant something to me.' So we made a difference in two families' lives," Monica said. That summer Christian and Monica also organized several day-long rafting trips for reservists from the Calgary Highlanders and their families. "We couldn't really measure what it did for them, being outdoors together with their families and with their comrades, back from combat," said Monica. "But they knew they felt better, being outside, being in the fresh air, being in the water as cold as it was, just made them feel good. We knew we were on the right track."[3]

The CVAF spent the next year and a half solidifying itself as a non-profit organization; it ran its next weekend-long program for veterans from the Saskatoon OSI clinic in August 2009. The participants, all veterans who had served in the Canadian Forces in various locations including the Balkans, Somalia and Haiti, and all of whom were suffering from post-traumatic experiences, arrived on a Friday night to a campsite that Christian had set up in Kananaskis Country, a provincial park approximately an hour west of Calgary. Also accompanying the group were Dr. Susan Brock, the leader of the Saskatoon OSI clinic, and Dr. Greg Passey, a psychiatrist who works with veterans in Vancouver.

Saturday involved a full day of rafting—on the Bow River in the morning and the Kananaskis River in the afternoon. Saturday night, all the participants returned to the campsite for dinner and sat around the campfire for the evening, talking and reminiscing. On Sunday, the group took a trip into the mountain town of Banff, including visits to Bow Falls and the Banff Hot Springs. "After the first river in the morning on Saturday, you could see the guys melting, starting to relax and smile and have a little bit of fun," Christian remembered, "They were quite happy that they could be successful at something again."

Ian Sherrington, who was also on the trip, similarly reflected that "you could see life flowing back into [the veterans] over the two and a half days that we had them, and at the end, they were all completely charged." Ian said, "You could see the benefits—you didn't need to be a sociologist or a psychologist to see it, it was just there." In the end, Monica reported that the weekend was "a big success," telling me, "We measure it as a success because the guys who came measured it as a success—that's the important factor."

The success of the weekend was backed by several participant testimonials posted on the CVAF's website.[4] For example, one participant wrote: "It's nice to feel like part of the team again. As a serving member with PTSD you don't feel like part of the team and sometimes because of the way PTSD affects us we are treated like and told…we aren't part of the team, and then we are released which rips us from the team. Christian, Monica, Ian and board of directors, thank you for the new team." Another participant shared that "it was the most fun, most relaxed, the first time in a long time that most of us weren't angry, worried, on guard or overwhelmed…I actually felt important, that I wasn't forgotten and that someone actually cared how I felt."

Psychiatrist Dr. Greg Passey wrote the following:

> The CVAF program provides a rare opportunity for Veterans with physical and OSI type injuries to engage in outdoor activities that they may have otherwise thought they were incapable of doing. The variety of special Canadian natural settings and adventure activities that the CVAF uses can provide a calming effect and a sense of peace in veterans that are often struggling on a day to day basis. CVAF provides a safe environment with a focus on the activity of the day. This encourages interaction with other veterans with similar health issues which helps to diminish their sense of isolation and difficulty connecting to others. The sharing of their current and past experiences in this type of environment can form an important part of their healing/recovery process. Having experienced it first hand and witnessing the positive effect it had on all the participating veterans, it is a program that I would recommend.[5]

Christian emphasized the importance of the camaraderie that developed over the weekend amongst the veterans, many of whom did not know one another, or who had only met at their group therapy sessions. Both the participants' and Dr. Passey's comments highlighted the same benefit.

Sitting around the campfire with the other veterans after the day of rafting, Christian said, "It's probably one of the first times that I've sat around with a group of army guys who had a good time when alcohol wasn't involved." By about 10:00 PM, as the veterans' talk around the campfire turned to the topic of war and their involvement in the former Yugoslavia, Christian recalled that several of the participants were "starting to trigger a bit—the 'fucks' started coming out and the swear words and all that kind of stuff." But despite increased tension and "edginess" within the group, Christian said that unlike an indoor therapy setting, "it was really easy to diffuse it because everybody was having a good time."

The presence of tension and negative energy are something that Christian has thought about often in his own life. He has personally noticed that when he grooms his horse while talking about incidents or events related to his military service, "it just takes the edge off it a little bit and makes it a lot easier to talk about and doesn't have that lasting effect. Normally guys can get ramped up [in indoor therapy settings], and they'll stay that way for days, so that's one of the benefits about the outdoors." Further, Christian told me, "I've done a lot of thinking about the energy that's involved with trauma and trying to get people going, and my theory has been that sitting with a group of guys that are angry in a room with nowhere for all that energy to go isn't always helpful." He recalled how rather than reducing his anger, such group therapy sessions have often led him to feel angrier than he was before the session. Christian continued, "One of the things I began to ask when I was on that expedition [on the Columbia River] was 'Why does group therapy have to be in an office or a clinical situation? What's wrong with having a group of guys talking about the same traumatic stuff around a campfire after a day of canoeing, or something like that?' With being outside, that energy has a place to go."

In August 2010, the CVAF ran a second successful mountain retreat for the veterans from Saskatoon who had attended the previous summer. Then, in July 2011, just as the organization really seemed to be getting its feet and had planned a variety of programs for veterans, the CVAF disbanded due to a lack of funding; however, based on his personal experiences, Christian has continued to advocate for the importance of nature for all people. "There are benefits across the board for everybody, whether they're healthy or they're totally sick." He noted specifically for veterans that "what works for one doesn't always work for somebody else," and observed that while "the medications and the doctors are key, it's not the only thing that will help the vet move forward."

In the past decade, Christian believes that his relationships with his dogs and his horses have been of primary importance, to the point that he said, "for me having my animals has replaced people literally." In early 2013, his long-time dog Nevada died. Nevada, Christian recalled "was there when I was just getting released out of the army, in the dark days. And he was my support structure. If I could put one thing on what has kept me alive, it was my dog. I didn't want to leave him behind." Christian is a strong believer in service dogs. "Dogs give you something to live for, responsibility for something other than yourself, so you have to get up in the morning. Even if you don't want to face the world, they're sitting there waiting." He still misses Nevada a lot, and said that the therapeutic connection the two shared is not necessarily there with his two

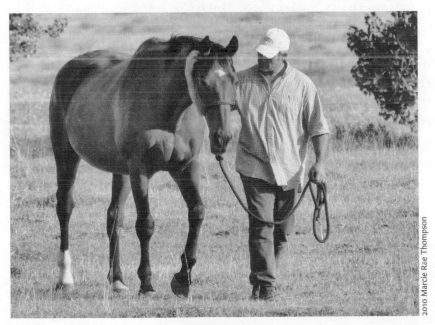

2010 Marcie Rae Thompson

Christian McEachern and his horse Sozo

other dogs, Nakoda and Buddy. "I think the relationship has now been replaced by my horses," he told me.

In 2007, Monica rescued a Thoroughbred gelding and ex-racehorse named Sozo, who was having difficulty adjusting to life after racing and was destined for slaughter. But despite Monica's efforts, Sozo would not bond with her; Christian, meanwhile, was visiting Sozo every day in the pasture, just to say hello. He described, "We were a little bit clashy at first, but he ended up taking to me." And so Monica eventually gave Christian the reins, and said, "Looks like you've got your first horse." Christian added, "I always think it's funny, the way Monica describes my first horse: 'Veteran racehorse with a problem with authority and PTSD meets army veteran with PTSD and a problem with authority.'" In fact, Christian observed, there are many similarities between ex-racehorses and military veterans. Just like veterans, ex-racehorses "did something hardcore at a high pace for so long, and all of a sudden they're not in a glamorous world anymore. Quite often they're thrown away after racing, so a lot of them have problems with authority, trust and relationships."

Christian's face lit up when I asked about Sozo's name. "He's got a racing history and I don't know what it is, but the name that he came to us with was Sozo." The name means "to heal." And the bond and trust that developed between Sozo and Christian has been healing for both. Monica described important changes that came about from Christian's relationship with Sozo. "I've certainly seen a difference in Christian since he got his horse. He's a lot more grounded, he's a lot more cognizant of his own behavior. He thinks about something else first instead of himself; he has to put that creature first."

It took a while for Christian to notice the effect that horses were having on him. "I don't know if it really hit me for a couple of years," he said. "It's just crept up on me over time, and it's gotten more and more powerful." Not long after getting Sozo, Christian got a second horse, a large black Percheron/Thoroughbred-cross mare named Charme, whom he rescued when she was five-months old. Christian described raising her and then beginning to ride her as "the completion of a cycle." Christian admitted, "It was one of the coolest things I've done in my life—and I have some pretty cool things under my belt—but it was just really cool to be able to ride her and share that time with her after having raised her."

Looking back over the past six years, Christian laughed as he realized how much his life had changed. He remembered how in 2007, when he and Monica were getting ready to put the CVAF horse-drawn wagon into the Calgary Stampede parade, "they had to take me kicking and screaming for a cowboy hat, Wranglers and cowboy boots into Lammle's [a Western wear and tack store]. I hated everything country." That was shortly before Sozo came into his life. Five years later, Christian spent a year working on a ranch in southern Alberta and found that he'd gone from hating everything cowboy to loving it. "How the hell did I end up here?" he wondered. "And I love it! It's a fantastic lifestyle. I'd love to have my own ranch, but it's just so expensive to get into; with the prices, it's impossible to get started unless you already have family that has a place."

Because horses mirror the emotions we bring when we're around them, Christian told me, "I've learned how to focus myself and leave my emotions at the gate when I'm working with horses." And he expressed the importance of being in the present moment with a horse: "There's a peace that you can't really explain when you're with them." In addition to being aware of the surroundings and the horse's personality, current mood and what the horse is communicating so that you don't get hurt, said Christian, "You really have to be in the moment with the horses, and I think that helps a lot. I tend not to think about everything that's going on when I'm in my zone with them."

Christian confessed that he likely would not have been in the right frame of mind to accept horses into his life when he first got out of the Forces. "It's a peace that I wouldn't have been able to accept ten years ago when I was really angry. That's not the right place to be when you're with horses. But I think they came to me at a time when I was ready for them." And he described ways that he has seen other veterans' personal walls also come down more easily while spending time with horses. He recalled how, during the 2009 CVAF program when the veteran participants came out to his place near Priddis, "car doors were still open and dinging, with keys in the ignition, and the guys were lined up at the

fence with the horses. It was really cool to see." Christian and his partner Marcie recently participated in an equine-therapy weekend through
Can Praxis[6] outside of Rocky Mountain House, where he similarly noticed the important ways that horses help bring down emotional walls.
Christian was particularly excited about Can Praxis's focus on families,
which is something that he had planned to incorporate into the CVAF
as well. "Families really do suffer as much as, if not more than, anybody
else."

When we last spoke, Christian was renting a house with Marcie on a
small acreage southwest of Calgary, just outside the small town of Black
Diamond. He had six horses, five of which are rescues. He bought his
sixth horse, a Dutch Warmblood/Andalusian cross named Pachino,
because he wanted to learn to do some jumping. When I asked if he
rides every day, Christian replied, "Oh yeah, I try to." Most often, he
rides either Charme or Pachino. Sozo injured his leg in 2009, and while
Christian does ride him on occasion, he is mindful that Sozo's healed
leg is no longer as strong as it once was and could easily be re-injured
in a more permanent way that would affect the horse's quality of life. In
the next few years, Christian is hoping to grow the number of horses in
his herd to eight or ten. He intends to start his own guiding business,
taking small groups on trail rides into the mountains. "It seems everything now is falling onto my horse plate; it's where I'm supposed to be.
I don't know what it's going to look like yet." When I asked if he'll ever
work with other veterans again, he was unsure. "I'd like to be helping
vets—that's what I was really good at. Am I going to get back there? I
don't know, we'll see."

5

Tangible Results

Penny Dex, Doug Fir Veterans
and Boots to Roots

*Penny Dex served as a pharmacy technician in the US Army from 2004
to 2008, during which time she was the victim of military sexual trauma
(MST). Inspired by the Veterans' Sanctuary, Penny and a group of friends
founded Doug Fir Veterans and its farm program, Boots to Roots, as an outreach project for veterans.*[1]

🌿 🌿 🌿

Penny Dex recalled her chance meeting with the founder of the Portland chapter of Iraq Veterans Against the War (IVAW) at a May Day
rally in 2011. Before that day, she said, "I didn't know there was such a
thing as pro-soldier, anti-war vets." It was also the first time she was addressed as a veteran. To that point, Penny didn't even consider herself
to be a veteran because she was female, had never deployed and had
worked in a hospital for all her time in the military. Even her parents
didn't consider her to be a veteran. "I wasn't a hero," she had concluded.
"I just put pills in a bottle and made IVs."

Penny served as a pharmacy technician in the US Army from 2004
until 2008, when she left with an honorable discharge. However, when
she left the military, Penny left with something else: post-traumatic
stress from military sexual trauma (MST). She was raped twice while
in the military, but when she reported the rapes to her superiors, she

was threatened with ostracization and retaliation. While still serving, in an attempt to manage her profound sensation of being targeted and overwhelmed, she sought out mental health counseling; but rather than supporting her, other soldiers were warned not to spend time with her.

"She's just trying to cause trouble; she's not a good soldier; she's just trying to get out of work by going to all these mental health appointments," were some of the comments Penny heard during that time. And rather than having her experiences of sexual trauma acknowledged, Penny was told that she had a personality disorder. "They said that after four years in the military, I just couldn't hack it. I just couldn't adapt to military life, so obviously I had a personality disorder going in," she recalled. This response has left Penny with what she described as a chip on her shoulder. "Having the whole stigma that there's something wrong with me, that if I'd just kept my mouth shut, I could have had a career," she said, her disbelief clear.

Based on these experiences, once she left the military in 2008, Penny was reluctant to go to the VA for help and to have her MST acknowledged. At that time, she told me, only about ⅓ of MST-related PTSD claims were getting approved. "The rest were told, 'nope, not enough evidence, didn't happen'. And to have to go through the whole thing of bringing all that stuff up and getting testimonies, and then to have the government tell you once again that you're just making it up, it's fake, it's not legitimate—that can really set a lot of people off. It can be a really bad trigger and make those who were traumatized never want to go to the VA again. So I was putting it off, and putting it off and putting it off."

Then, in 2013, the US federal law changed. Victims of MST, rather than being required to provide detailed documentation of their assault, could now be assessed by a psychiatrist. With that, Penny said, "I finally got up the courage to go try." She made the appointment in early 2013 and received her PTSD rating on May 8, 2013. When I asked what the rating means to her, she said it's bittersweet: "It feels good to finally be acknowledged. It's been a long process, and this is just the diagnosis. I haven't gotten anything saying whether it was service connected or not. That's a whole other process I have to go through, and God knows how long that will take."

For a long time, Penny avoided people and situations that reminded her of her trauma. Today, she is more willing to talk about her experience, although "it's really hard saying it out loud," she admitted. For example, during a recent public talk about her organization, Doug Fir Veterans, the topic of MST came up. "None of the people in the room knew what MST was, so then it turned into an hour-long talk on MST," she recalled. "Afterward, I just wanted to go home and die. It was cathartic and horrible at the same time, because it brought up all this stuff in me that I haven't dealt with for the past five years." Prior to that, she believes her veteran activism helped conceal her symptoms. Most of that work was with male combat veterans. She said, "I really did not want to deal with female vets, because their stories would remind me just how hard my time in the Army was. At first I thought it was just a bunch of personality conflicts, and I that I didn't want to be around those issues; but then I realized that those issues are my issues, and I didn't want to be around it because every time other women talked about their military sexual trauma or rape or sexual assault, it would trigger all this emotion in me and I would get angry, I would get set off again. But now I finally took that step and acknowledged it, and I'm going to go through the whole process."

🍃 🍃 🍃

Like many veterans who leave the military and experience difficulty finding work, despite her years spent as a pharmacy technician in the Army, Penny was unable to obtain work in a civilian pharmacy because she didn't have civilian certifications and experience. She was living in Centralia, Washington, at the time, a small town on the I5. After almost a year, she did find work, but quickly became frustrated and disenchanted with the realities of a civilian pharmacy. "I never had to deal with insurance in the military," Penny said. "I never knew what the actual prices of the medications were, because in the military you just give that stuff out like candy. You don't have to worry about whether people are going to get denied. The DoD just gives medication to them. I never knew that people were paying $300 a bottle for their cholesterol medication. I didn't know you could deny a kid his asthma medication because they were two days early on it, even though he was having an asthma attack right in your lobby."

Penny also became frustrated by the food choices available to people in her community, which she saw as contributing to many of the health problems that needed treating. "The place where I lived, it's all Walmart, McDonald's, Subway, a lot of corporate stuff, and people were just eating garbage all the time," she observed. "It just really bothered me on a fundamental level: these people were treating the symptoms of their problems, but if they just went out and exercised and had a better diet, they probably wouldn't have all these health problems." Eventually, Penny quit her job and moved to Portland, Oregon, where she started pursuing a degree in biology at Washington State University (WSU) across the state border in Vancouver, Washington.

"At that point, I wasn't into veterans' activism. I didn't really have any veteran friends," she recalled. "I was just trying to get back into school, get on with my life." And Portland provided a stark contrast to the conservative mindset in Centralia. "We have a hundred-some community-supported agriculture programs within the city limits. Our farmer's market is one of the best in the world. And people are just healthier down here. They don't have the same rates at the pharmacy. They have naturopaths and acupuncturists, and people believe more in holistic care; I got really interested in that. But I wasn't sure how to make all these connections."

When she began her studies at WSU, Penny still planned to become a pharmacist, but along the way she realized, "I didn't want to be just one more pill pusher in the world. I wanted to treat the root of problems." As she became involved in veteran activism through IVAW, Penny began to understand the difficulties facing other veterans, both in Oregon and throughout the country. Oregon, Penny explained, has the highest veteran suicide rate of any other state in the US, despite the fact that it has no active-duty military bases. One-third of the homeless population in Portland are veterans, and many of the female veterans were sexually assaulted in the military (approximately one in three female veterans nation-wide were victims of MST).[2] There is also high unemployment amongst female veterans living in Oregon.

"What my generation is dealing with is being homeless, being unemployed, their job experience not transferring," Penny told me. Friends who were combat medics in Afghanistan had similar experiences to her own of trying to find work. "They did their job in Afghanistan, taking care of everything from heavy trauma to light bruises and scrapes, and then they come home and they can't even be a school nurse because they don't have the proper certifications. They just get very discouraged. Then they have to go find a new job and train for that, and that costs money; and trying to jump into a school environment right after deployment is not very productive. So even though we have the G.I. Bill, if vets don't have a support group and a network that they can rely on and help relieve stress and help identify with, they don't do very well."

Through IVAW, Penny became involved in organizing and attending marches, rallies and protests about the war. But then the Iraq War ended. "And it's like, 'well, shit, what do we do now?'" Penny told me. "People are still dying, people are still committing suicide. More soldiers lost their lives through suicide in 2009, 2010 and 2011 than did in combat. So things are still bad, and we didn't know what to do." Eventually, she decided to focus at the grassroots level. "There are at least 50,000 vets in Multnomah County. How are we going to help them?"

Penny, along with several other veterans, initially planned to open a pro-soldier, anti-war coffee shop called The Grounds for Resistance, which would be a community space where veterans and civilians could find common ground over coffee. Any money raised would go to funding other veteran projects. The group took business classes and worked hard on a business plan. Penny recalled the pride she felt showing that plan to a Vietnam veteran and small business manager at the local community college, and her surprise at his angry response: "He's like, 'Why the hell are you doing this?' And I said, 'I want to help build a community space. And I want to help veterans get jobs.' He's like, 'Well, the last thing that people when they get out of the military want to deal with is bullshit. Why are you creating a place where all they're going to have to deal with is bullshit?'"

In hindsight, Penny understood his reaction. She explained to me, "If you have any idea what the coffee culture is in Portland, it's every stereotype you see on TV. People are really snotty about it, and why would I take a bunch of combat infantry people and put them behind a counter, having to make people in skinny jeans a half-decaf split shot macchiato?" She laughed.

"Then he said, 'What do you want to do with the money that you raise from this?' And I said, 'Well, we heard of this Veterans' Sanctuary they have out in Ithaca, New York. We want to be able to raise money to buy a farm.'" The small business manager looked at her and asked, "Why don't you just do that? It takes just as much planning to do something big as it does something small. If you're going to waste all this energy, you might as well put it toward something productive." So, they sat down to write a new business plan to buy a farm where veterans could come to work and spend time, and that's how the Veterans' Transition Corps—reorganized as Doug Fir Veterans in 2013—and its farm program, Boots to Roots, was born.

"Veterans want to do this," Penny explained. "When they get out in the dirt and they get out in the grass—I have guys who can't sleep in the city, they'll be up for three days at a time. But if you take them out to the farm, you give them a sleeping bag, they curl up on the ground and they will snore like logs." The ultimate goal, she explained, would be to pay the veterans while they're doing this work. At the same time, there are other veterans who have 100% disability ratings and just need something to do. "They need a purpose," said Penny. "And working on a farm helps them find that."

Moreover, on the farm, military training and even some of the symptoms associated with post-traumatic stress can be turned to veterans' advantage. "When people describe PTSD in the States, it's seen as making you a ticking time bomb waiting to go off against the uncaring system that created you," Penny told me. "But I see it as a perk—that hypervigilance, that always ready to do something, always needing to pull security. On the farm, it really works because if you have holes in the fence, you need to make sure that all the animals are squared away; that attention to detail is important."

⊕ ⊕ ⊕

During her childhood, Penny recalled, "any house where we got to have animals or we got to grow food was one of the better places to live." Growing up in an apartment in southern California did not lend itself to gardening in her early life, and then with yearly moves for her father's work from the time she was seven, gardening was not a priority. But Penny's mother had grown up in rural Texas—"living on a homestead until she was twelve"—and so when the family moved to Durham, California where they would stay for two years, Penny's mom announced, "This year we're going to have a garden!" She brought soil in because the quality of the dry butte land in the area was not conducive to growing anything. "My dad was furious!" recalled Penny. "She paid $700 to have all this dirt trucked in so that she could grow potatoes. And my dad relished his $700 potatoes! Then we ended up getting emus as well, and we got to have dogs to guard the emus, and it became a little homestead."

When the family moved to Dry Ridge, Kentucky, Penny was awed by the landscape. "Growing up in California, I'd never seen people who had acres and acres of just grass and yards." There, the family got bees, and the kids joined 4H and started raising chickens. At first Penny didn't understand why they were doing these things. "I was so consumer-from-Southern California brainwashed, and thought, we can just go to the store! Why would you raise these things that can sting you? Once I got stung in the arm 11 times, and I was not thrilled with the whole apiary thing."

In high school, her family moved to Washington State where they kept goats and sheep. Penny and her siblings enrolled in Future Farmers of America (FFA). "That's how my mom wanted to get us socialized," Penny said. "We ended up raising 25 chickens—those genetically altered fryer chickens—that basically go from chick to adult bird in 6 weeks." With her passion for biology, Penny was at first excited when she learned about genetic engineering. But those chickens made her think differently. "All they did was eat and poop. And we had them in this chicken tractor, which is like a cage that you move around on the grass so they're not always in one area. And you'd move them a foot and they would be limping and fall over and look like they were going to die, because all of their energy went to making breast meat! We got them at one or two weeks old, and they grew so fast their legs would snap under the weight of their chests." When she got the chicks, Penny worried about her ability to butcher them, but by the end of six weeks, she saw it as a mercy killing. "That was my first jaunt into 'this is not how things are supposed to be.'"

While in high school, Penny enrolled in the Washington State Running Start program which enables high-school students in their junior year to take community college classes. By the time she graduated in 2004, Penny had both her high-school diploma and a two-year community college degree. From there, she joined the military. She completed boot camp at Leonard Wood in Missouri, and then a ten-week advanced individual training program in Texas. For the next four years, she served as a pharmacy technician at Reynolds Army Community Hospital in Lawton, Oklahoma. Penny reflected on the cultural differences between her life in Portland and her time in Oklahoma: "Here in Portland, people take eating healthy to an extreme. Out in Oklahoma, they take it to the other extreme, as in 'how quickly can I meet Jesus by eating food?'" Fast food outlets provided the majority of food options around the army base, and it was nearly impossible to find fresh produce, so by her second year there, Penny was driving three hours to a farmer's market in Dallas, Texas.

⊕ ⊕ ⊕

Penny points to small-scale agriculture as one way that veterans can engage in healing sensory activities. While she and other veterans can find themselves stuck in "that tunnel vision of depression, where nothing in the world makes sense anymore," she said, "when you get on the farm, when you're pruning, when you're doing things old school—you're out there digging and shovelling and putting in a fence line and having to cut and do all these tactile things, added with the sensation of touching the animals—it helps get out of that whole internal self-focusing. You realize that there are other things to see, that there are other things beside yourself going on in the world. And it's a pretty awesome sensation!"

And while Penny hasn't experienced difficulties with the triggers of an urban enviroment, she knows veterans who have. "With PTSD, a lot of the people can't be in the city. I know one guy who starts vomiting every time he smells gasoline because he's been in so many IED attacks," she said. "So getting veterans out to the farm gets them away from that, and it calms them down immensely. It takes away so many stressors. It takes away so many variables because they can see five acres in every direction. They know what's going on. And there's just not as much stuff to deal with. You have a routine out on the farm. You get up, you feed the goats, you feed the chickens, you take the hay from here to there," she explained. "You get to see the results of your labor. Whatever work you put into it, you get out of it. Yes, there can still be variables. There can still be all kinds of things that happen, like a frost comes too early or pests start eating your crops. But when you're working together as a team, you figure out how to fix that."

Boots to Roots, Doug Fir Veterans' farm program, has worked on projects on two properties for the past two years. One is a five-acre wooded property in Oregon City owned by a veteran who served in the military for 22 years, who "wanted to grow his own food, be off the grid a little bit, have something he could sell at the farmer's market like a little side business while he's doing his day job, so we helped set up his property for that." The entire focus is permaculture, making the farm ideal for veterans who are triggered by city noises, smells and crowds. "There are no gasoline tools whatsoever, except an occasional chainsaw," Penny explained. "A lot of our guys will take that extra step because they don't want to use petroleum products—they would find it ironic to be using petroleum on a veterans' sanctuary. They just want to go back to using the manual tools, learning some skills that way."

It was on that property in Oregon City that Boots to Roots ran its first two-week pilot program in 2012. As far as Penny knows, the course was the "first veteran-run, veteran-taught permaculture design course" in the US. Initially, 20 veterans signed up, but many backed out at the last minute and only 8 committed to the course full-time. Those 8 helped turn a 4,000-square-foot blackberry patch into a permaculture garden with raised beds, its own fertilizer system, a rabbit hutch, herb spiral and a keyhole garden. Doug Fir Veterans continues to be involved on that property, using its network to scour the Internet for supplies, such as chicken wire, two-by-fours, saws and other resources to help on the farm.

The other property is Brookside Farm, a small five-acre hobby farm on the Portland city limits with laying hens, goats, beehives, apple, plum and walnut trees and blackberry bushes. The owners are an elderly couple, no longer able to keep up with the day-to-day requirements of the farm, who need help pruning trees, cleaning out chicken coops and other farm maintenance. Boots to Roots' dream is to eventually take over the property and create the first veterans' farm in Portland, which would be set up as a cooperative, where veterans could live, work and pay a certain amount per month to become equal shareholders in the farm. "There is nothing else like it in Oregon State, not that we've found yet, anyway," Penny said. The property, which is on a bus line, is also easily accessible for other veterans who have jobs or family or attend school.

When Penny and her team first took the farming idea to the City of Portland, officials expressed concern. Penny recalled them asking, "So this is a halfway house kind of thing, right?" to which she responded that it was not. "Well, are you going to allow drugs and alcohol on the property?" they asked, and Penny replied, "Not anymore than is in anybody else's house." City officials told her, "Well, you can't have that many people living in this place unless you're family, you're married or you're disabled."

"Well, hot damn! Guess what? All my guys have a disability rating— so technically we count as a family," Penny replied. Initially, the City was going to charge a $30,000 fee to consider—and not even necessarily ap- prove—the project. "But once we pulled the disabled family card, they decided to give us a $400 zoning certification fee. So we've gotten the green light from the City. Now we're just trying to figure out what kind of plan it would take to purchase the property outright."

In 2013, Doug Fir Veterans began selling the farm's eggs, both online and on street corners, which gets the veterans out in the community. "It gets people talking to them about something besides the war. It gets them seen as a valuable member—'Hey, that's the egg guy, I can feed my whole family on farm fresh eggs for a week because of this guy'—

and helps give them a new purpose." The veterans are also using the farm as a base for making value-added products. For example, Penny is making shrub, a drinking vinegar made with apple-cider vinegar, fruit and honey. Another veteran is making his own ketchups, mustards and barbeque sauces, another is making soap and another hot sauce, all of which they plan to sell at farmer's markets under the Doug Fir Veterans name. As a hobby farm, Brookside Farm is set up for all these ventures, including equipment (a tractor, various food processing machines and a cider press) and storage space. And in making these products, the members of Doug Fir Veterans are working to show various funding organizations that, as Penny said, "we are veterans with good heads on our shoulders; we want to be part of creating things from these products, showing people why we want to have local products." In addition, the group is once again working on a business plan, and gaining sales experience. They are also getting financial coaching from one of the farm's owners, who was once the president of a credit union. In partnership with her, the veterans are learning how to market themselves and their products.

All the hard manual labor at the farm has many benefits. "If you have to do it all by hand, at the end of the day, you're not stressing anymore," Penny explained. "I've known people that have been able to get off their Valium and their Ambien, their anti-anxiety meds and their insomnia aids, because they'd just go outside and work. They get tired again. They haven't been tired since they were in the Army." Penny also feels encouraged that many other veterans across the country "have already come to this conclusion and they're doing it on small scales, whether it's in their backyard or going out to the plethora of farms that we have here."

She told me the story of one veteran she met, who owned a house in Vancouver, Washington. He drank heavily upon returning from overseas, was apprehended by the police for driving while intoxicated and given an ankle bracelet. "We knew he had guns and stuff, and since he didn't have anything to do at his house, we brought him some blackberry bushes, raspberry bushes, some strawberries," Penny remembered. "He was all mad, and you know, 'fuck it, I'm not going to do this, blah, blah, blah,' and being all angry. But after a while we came back. We looked over the yard, and we would see these were planted. And then we would see that he had dug out a little irrigation ditch around it. And then we would see that he started a compost pile on the side. And after awhile, it got him through until his next court date. By that time he said, 'Yeah, maybe I should come out and help on the farm. It'd be fun. I tried doing this with the raspberries, what would you do?' That was one of our success stories."

⊕ ⊕ ⊕

After running its permaculture course, the Veterans Transition Corps began its evolution to Doug Fir Veterans. "When we became the Veterans Transition Corps, we had the idea that we were going to be a non-profit, have an executive director, and file with the IRS," said Penny. Their vision was of an organization committed to alternative treatments and supporting veterans who had fallen through the cracks of the VA system. Although Penny saw the group's August 2012 course as a success, some of the other members believed they'd failed when only 8 of the 20 veterans who signed up came out. Disillusioned, some of the others no longer wanted to go through the lengthy process of becoming a non-profit.

At that point, the veterans also recognized that they were not in a position to offer themselves as a treatment program, Penny explained, since most group members were dealing with their own post-military traumas. Some of the original members left, and the remaining members realized, "We're just local veterans wanting to make our community a better place, still wanting to serve our community in different means." In addition, because there are already more than 300 military non-profits in Oregon, they decided that they might be better off to become a network of veterans—"a local veteran community, that even if we couldn't help people directly address their issues, we know the places to refer them," said Penny. "We can give them the phone number so they'll actually have a person at the end of the line. We can give them a ride to where that person is and make sure that they actually see that person. And so we went from being a non-profit to a network that now includes about 50 veterans across Oregon and the Pacific Northwest, and we've decided to call ourselves Doug Fir Veterans because in Oregon, the Doug Fir is our state tree. It's basically a symbol of pride here." Veterans in the network assume responsibility for one another. "We hold ourselves accountable to make sure that everybody gets through the day."

Penny also realized the need to be more succinct about the group's goals. "It was my mistake last time to let the guys run with it because I was just so excited that they were participating," she observed. With new group members, including an equal number of women and men, Doug Fir Veterans began to focus on building the foundational groundwork of its organization, which includes taking more training and marketing courses. "I want to have a structured plan that everybody can see and agree to before branching out and doing things. Right now, with the whole network system, it's just about keeping people's heads above water. If someone needs a ride to the VA, we give them a ride to the VA. We help them get groceries, we stay up till two in the morning listening to each other going through whatever is going on in our minds. I'm really focusing more on building the community and the relationships in the group, versus trying to grab all these members and making ourselves out to be this big thing, when in actuality we're just a big group

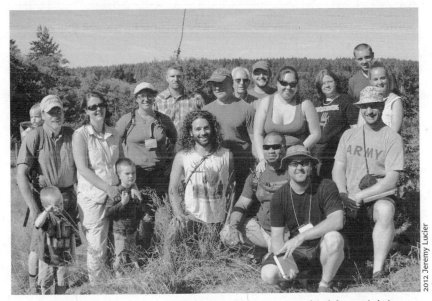

2012 Jeremy Lucier

The Doug Fir Veterans crew, with Penny Dex (top row, third from right)

of friends trying to show people how self-resiliency can be beneficial to the community."

While she admitted that the process is slower than she would like, Penny knows that, in the long run, a strong foundation will help Doug Fir Veterans achieve its goals. "I think that actually building the foundation, getting everything in writing, getting the business plans done, getting the help of the larger organizations that have been doing this for a while, it's a much better process."

Doug Fir Veterans' overall focus is post-9/11 veterans—anyone who served from September 2001 onwards. "We're all in our 20s to early 30s, and we're dealing with a lot of issues," Penny reflected. "By the time I find people, they already have a ton of credit card debt, they've been unemployed for the past six months or they've flunked out of school and they're frustrated about going back. We have a lot of trust issues as well." When veterans first joined the military, most "had all these ideals and they thought they were going to go be heroes, and then they actually get over there doing these things and they find that's not true. And they get back and they try to talk to civilians about their stuff, it's all, 'thank you for your service.' As one of my compatriots likes to say, 'If I had done over here what I did over there, would you be thanking me?' These vets end up getting really closed off and really isolated."

The isolation and difficulties experienced by these young veterans points to the importance of Doug Fir Veterans' work to find and reach out to the veterans in the community. "There are 50,000 vets in Multnomah County, and more than 6,000 of them are post 9/11," Penny told me, "And you have to dig for them. They're not on Facebook. They don't hang out in the mall. A lot of them just sit at home with their X-Box, and they're angry. They're really angry! They don't want to participate in the society that has rejected them or that doesn't make sense to them anymore. It's making those house calls that counts."

As with many other veterans' organizations, one of Doug Fir Veterans' biggest challenges is funding. "I'm finding out you do need a day job for these things," Penny explained. And based on her own difficulties trying to secure work, she told me, "There's a strong discriminatory leaning toward hiring people that have military experience, whether they've deployed or not. Everyone has this whole stigma that we're just this bunch of ticking time bombs, waiting to go off."

Penny recalled one interview at a coffee shop, when the interviewer asked if she'd ever killed anyone. "And if I was getting this question," she said, "then anybody who had 'veteran' on their fucking resume was getting that question." She told me later, "And it's really hard. How can you be a hero but also be feared? That's why we feel that having a farm run by vets for vets is really important, having veterans here that can actually help identify and talk people through this stuff and just let them know, hey, you're not crazy for thinking this. It's OK, there are lots of us that do. It's all right. There's nothing wrong with you."

Penny recently took the word veteran off her resume, and as soon as she did, she said, "I went from having no interviews or even phone calls for months to having four set up that week. It was ridiculous. I can't validate this, all I can do is offer an anecdotal story, but honest to God, that's what happened." She now works part-time at a doggy daycare, and the irony, she admitted, is that after taking veteran off her resume, she was hired for the job because she is a veteran. One of the daycare's previous best employees had been a US Navy veteran, so when the owners found out in the interview that Penny was a veteran, they thought she might be perfectly suited to the job. "But basically any other place where it came up that I was a vet, I didn't get a call back, even though I told them I didn't deploy, even though I worked in a pharmacy, that I never once held a weapon except for boot camp and training. They still see it as a liability."

In her current work, Penny's hypervigilance is beneficial. "You're always on guard, you're always aware, you're always looking out for things going on," she explained. "I have 50 dogs in a room, and I always have to be on the lookout to see if one of them is going to bite another one, if one of them is getting into something it shouldn't, and the owners really value that. But if there hadn't been a veteran working there before to show them why that is such a good thing to have, it would have scared them. Not a lot of people see that as an asset."

☙ ☙ ☙

Toward the end of one conversation, Penny reflected on the struggles that many veterans experience. "It's not so much that we're trying to integrate back into society, but rather that we want society to integrate back into us. We want society to understand that if you're going to send people to war for 11 years, they're not going to come back the same. They're not going to enjoy fireworks anymore. They're not going to be the same person they were before their multiple deployments." She emphasized that civilians should not be scared of veterans, but that veterans' experiences need to be better understood and respected. "A lot of these people, they can't talk to their family about this. They don't have the same support net after they leave the military. Everyone just tells them, 'Oh, you've changed so much when you get back.'"

In the end, it comes down to why vets joined the military in the first place. "We wanted to serve our country. We wanted to serve our communities," Penny said. And this desire to serve is still strong amongst many veterans. "We just want to do it the right way this time."

6

"We All We Got"

Deston Denniston and VETS_CAFE

Deston Denniston's US Army career was cut short by a head injury and spinal trauma sustained during a training accident. Twenty years later, these injuries crept back into his life to the point where he could no longer walk. Frustrated in his attempts to get compensation, Deston became permanently committed to veterans' issues. In 2012, he launched Veterans Entrepreneurial Training and Studies in Conservation Agriculture, Forestry and Ecology (VETS_CAFE) to work toward food security and local ecology initiatives for veterans, while also supporting them in building employment connections.[1]

"When we're engaged in our environment and we're out there in the garden or forest and we're listening to birds and we understand the soil granularity by touching it with our fingers, we're using more of our brain. This work expands our notions of who we are, and I think that's how we become full human beings," explained US Army veteran Deston Denniston, speaking about his experiences with gardening, farming and permaculture. Deston holds a clear vision of agriculture as looking "a lot more like an ecosystem than it does a farm" in contrast to large industrial farm systems. And he has been excited to find that an increasing number of veterans share his vision.

Deston spent his formative years in the 1970s and 1980s on small farms in southwest Washington, where he recalled reading old newsprint versions of *Mother Earth News* and tinkering in the wood shop. In his teens, many other young men around him were finding work in the timber industry, a place Deston imagined he'd end up too. But the mid-to-late-1980s saw a decline in the timber market, and jobs disappeared. For a while, Deston wandered "from one dish pit to another" in search of a more substantial career path, and in 1988, decided to enlist in the US Army.

After only two years, however, his military career was cut short by a training accident, in which Deston sustained a head injury and spinal trauma. He left the Army with an honorable discharge, and today looking back more than 20 years, Deston admitted: "When I got out of the Army, I was a mess. I'm just glad that I didn't have a combat situation to compound the confusion and outright madness that was my discharge. It took me seven years to get my first medical claim through." He received a 50% disability rating.

But Deston's dealings with the VA were far from over. By 2010, Deston could no longer walk. At the time, he was living on a small, isolated farm in southwest Washington State. Deston vividly recalled a moment of true despair when he found himself literally unable to get up off the ground. In that moment, Deston had the presence of mind to call a friend. "You know what?" he said. "This is *that* call. This is the call you don't want to get, but it's the one that's better than the call that you really don't want to get. Come and pick my ass up because I can't get it off the ground." Deston had several fully herniated discs, and doctors told him that that he'd been suffering from degenerative back issues since his accident in 1990. For the next month, Deston could not walk. And for another 4 months, he was only able to stand for about 20 minutes per day. It took nearly 23 years for the VA to process his medical claim for peripheral neuropathy, which was finally awarded in October 2013. His medical claim for traumatic brain injury (TBI) is still in process.

"I tried to get health care from the VA and was utterly confounded by the system," Deston told me; however, he was fortunate to have several friends who are health care providers outside the VA system; they helped him to recover some of his abilities. Today, while he continues to have numbness in his leg, Deston is able to perform most day-to-day tasks: walking, riding a bike and operating a chainsaw among other things. "Nobody could tell if they watched me walk that I was having problems." But Deston does feel challenged by his leg's numbness and the resulting uncoordination. While he would like to go back to studying martial arts, which he did for a number of years, he's not sure it would be safe: "I don't feel able to move gracefully and adeptly so that I can avoid being hurt and hurting others while I practice." He also described how, despite his 50% disability rating, when he was unable to walk, he could not even get a crutch from the VA, adding, "The VA didn't give me one single bit of help aside from pills. They would give me any pill I wanted. As much of them as I could take." But Deston didn't want pills. He was sure that if he had access to acupuncture, massage and neuropathic therapies he could increase his mobility and coordination, but these types of therapies are not available through the VA. "This is not good enough," Deston stated emphatically.

It was his distressing and frustrating experiences of trying to get assistance from the VA that led Deston to become permanently committed to veterans' issues. "I know for a fact that it's possible to have injuries and have all the records, all the documentation, to have submitted it multiple times, and to be denied the disability benefit multiple times." Deston's private doctors and doctors through the VA have examined both his Service Medical Records and his current medical data, and all agree that there is clear evidence that he suffers from a head injury. "Yet the VA loses the paperwork every time I submit it!" he told me. "I've been through two congressional inquiries, and they come back and say, 'You don't have a file. You don't have any medical records.' And I had them in my hand. I said, 'Here they are. Would you like to see them?' This is how broken the VA system is."

As he reflected on his own experience, Deston also began to think about the number of post-9/11 soldiers who would become veterans by 2017. Aware of the astounding rates of PTSD and TBI amongst this group, he turned his attention to how he might support other veterans experiencing similar frustrations. "I want to be in a place where my experience can serve their ability to transition into some kind of a livelihood where they are going to be able to access health care and there are going to be networks where their neighbors and their fellow veterans can give mutual aid to one another because the VA just doesn't cut it!" Deston added, "If nothing else, maybe I can help guide other veterans away from having to experience what I experienced because they've already got enough to deal with. I didn't have the disadvantages of coming back with the kind of mental and emotional wounding that goes on in combat."

And thinking back to that day when, unable to get off the ground, he made that desperate phone call to a friend, Deston said that he hopes to "steer somebody away from having to ever make that kind of a choice again and get them with some dirt under their fingernails."

⚘ ⚘ ⚘

Several years ago, Deston gathered with some other veterans to start a garden at a state-owned Veterans' Home in Orting, Washington. From 1880 to 1933, the Home had an operational farm where residents collectively shared the work. The Washington State VA owned 12 acres of land and leased another 80 acres, which enabled the veterans to plant orchards and also keep a herd of cows. "That farm produced so much food that the veterans couldn't eat it all, so they shared it with their community," Deston explained. But in 1934, "in the middle of the Great Depression, it was somehow or other deemed fiscally irresponsible to be feeding the community," Deston commented wryly. "The farm got shut down, and the veterans began to buy their food from other farms on a federal dole."

Nearly 80 years later, a group of veterans, which included Deston, submitted a project proposal to the Washington State VA so that veterans at the Home could once again grow vegetables on the former farm site and raise some laying hens as well. The plan was to start small, said Deston, "to produce enough vegetables to keep the kitchen in some fresh produce in season and get farm fresh eggs a couple days a week." Administrators at the VA Home were excited by the proposal, but there was a hitch: it had to go through the Department of Natural Resources (DNR), which held an interagency management contract on the now-fallow land. And DNR officials vetoed the project. "We didn't get to present our proposal. We didn't get to have a discussion about the needs that we were meeting in the community."

After six months of pressure, DNR officials relented and offered "a one-year memorandum of use," with terms that would see the DNR continuing to receive its regular land-management fee. But, as Deston pointed out, "You can't really farm on a year-to-year lease," so the group chose not to proceed with the project. And it was at that point that Deston decided to go freelance. "I was going to go out and I was going to find a veteran who owned land and say, 'How'd you like to bring a bunch of veterans here to help you farm? And we're going to teach them how to farm when we do that.' So I found a vet, and that's what we're doing."

⊛ ⊛ ⊛

Administrators at the Washington State Department of Veterans Affairs had been keen on starting a garden at the Veterans' Home in Orting, and so in 2012, they provided Deston with a monthly partnership stipend to develop Veterans Entrepreneurial Training and Studies in Conservation Agriculture, Forestry and Ecology (VETS_CAFE). "The State Veterans Affairs department is different than the Federal VA," explained Deston. "The state is often more able to work with veterans who have needs and able to find them resources even if they don't have them in their own docket." VETS_CAFE aims to work toward food security and local ecology initiatives for veterans, while also building community connections to help veterans find work.

Although he'd run programs through the regional permaculture network for about ten years, Deston ran his first veteran-specific program in conjunction with Boots to Roots in August 2012 in Oregon City. Then in 2013, he facilitated VETS_CAFE's first Winter Weekends Permaculture Design Course for eight veterans, which entailed designing a permaculture operation for a 2.5-acre veteran-owned farm in north-east Olympia. Through an arrangement with Evergreen State College, the participants received college credits for completing the program. Over six weekends from January to March, and with several optional fieldtrips, Deston brought in guest teachers, ranging from forestry specialists and energy systems designers to permaculture teachers and those with experience facilitating entrepreneurial ventures. Although the course had only 8 official participants, on some days, the workshops hosted up to 60 people. And many of the graduates continue to be interested and involved in

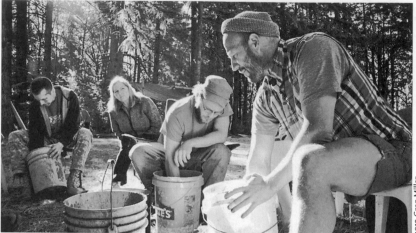

2012 Greg Miller

Deston Denniston (right) mixing seedballs during the 2012 permaculture course

permaculture in some way. "It's really interesting to see how tapping into this idea that we can live in a way that has lighter impact on the planet is something that I see veterans organizing in multi-generationally," Deston said. "I find that very exciting!"

For the duration of three months, the course participants also spent a lot of time discussing their experiences as veterans, which was important to building community amongst the group. Of the eight participants, five suffered from various degrees of post-traumatic stress. "All the combat vets had their PTSD show up at one point in time during the course," Deston told me. And several of the non-combat veterans also had "pretty intense military triggers while we were going through the course material and the site material."

Deston admitted that he qualifies as a "doubting Taoist" as to whether the programs he has run will lead to long-term prospects for veterans. "I'm really happy that I was able to give a reference and that one of my guys got a job," he said. "At the same time, it is only a nine-month internship. It's not going to allow him to save any money. He's not on his own farm, or working on a farm that he has an ownership stake in." Another veteran was so inspired by the August 2012 course that he walked onto a farm and announced his intentions to work for them; they couldn't turn him down. "He wants to be on the farm, and that's his life's passion now. He knew that he was interested in it before the course, but now he understands what capacity for healing and helping one's neighbor there is in being able to do this kind of work." But while Deston was happy that several of the participants have found opportunities, he admitted, "I want to see more—much more—access to land. And so much more real, enduring employment opportunity."

⊕ ⊕ ⊕

The difficulty of unemployment and under-employment facing many veterans is familiar to Deston, who commented, "I wouldn't by any means say that I'm making it right now." After graduating in 2000 with a dual BA/BSc in Ecological Design from Evergreen State College in Washington State, he spent several years following his passions and interests. "I spent a long time running around, working on different rural communities' infrastructure projects, building houses, putting in irrigation systems, figuring out how to grow food in places that were pretty dry without irrigation systems. And building straw bale houses and things like that."

Deston then completed a master's degree in 2007 from Washington State University with a major in ecological-agricultural-economics systems analysis and minor in rural and regional community planning, graduating *magna cum laude* (with high honors). However, despite applying for more than 200 jobs since 2006, he has had only three interviews. He worked odd jobs when he could find them and relied the rest of the time on the small disability payment he gets from the VA. He also grew a lot of his own food.

In 2003, Deston purchased a small, secluded farm in southwest Washington. He was deeply troubled when the US declared war on Iraq, but it wasn't until recently that he began wondering whether the timing of his farm purchase was coincidental. "And I've determined that it wasn't. I've gone back and read in my journals what I was writing, and even though I wouldn't say that I was a survivalist, I quit a job making $40,000 a year working part-time and fled to the hills. And I didn't recognize that that's what I was doing at the time, but now that I look back, that's exactly what I did."

When his previous military injuries became debilitating, however, Deston could no longer do the work required on the farm. At the time, he said, "I realized that I'd just spent a decade of my life living alone on a mountain top. It went by in a snap of the fingers. I don't even really know what I did up there other than eat and feed myself and put in a bunch of waterworks, and then I'd go travel around to different jobs when I could get them."

Deston sold his farm in 2013. "And now that I'm coming down from the mountain, I realize that I need people. I'm no longer young and really strong and able to survive and surmount all physical obstacles. And I need people. I gained a lot of self-sufficiency skills up there that are of interest to people. The one thing that I hope I gained the most was how to encourage other people to realize that we all need each other. I come down here, and I see how fragmented things are, even where people live next to each other. We've got a lot of work to do."

$$\oplus \; \oplus \; \oplus$$

Deston emphasizes agriculture, permaculture and conservation as key methods for building community connections. "We all eat, and as we look at our landscape and we begin to understand that we are participants in this landscape with an incredible diversity of other players— not just humans but animals and plants—designing landscapes in the permaculture method, understanding ecology and being involved in creating conservation movements and projects informs us not just at a human community level, but also of what it's like to be another creature or another plant on this planet. They're all impacted by what we do and by what their neighbors are doing, just the same as we are. And if we can understand this—I take this food in and I eat and I'm healthy; I do this work and I feel better because I've been outside; I communicate with my friends and I learn about the events in my community and the people in my community and the pulse of my community and then I also communicate with these plants and I begin to understand the patterns and the languages that constitute the natural environment—these things, I think, are all essential to being human," Deston said, adding, "Our bodies and our brains are hardwired to one another."

Over the years, Deston has realized he prefers activities and ways of working through problems that require whole body engagement, compared to solely intellectual pursuits. "I want to be involved in the whole process," he explained. "And I want to share and explore that process with a team. Our brains are connected to our body, and we effectively cut it off by sitting at a desk all day. I think that everybody who's ever done any soldiering, especially field soldiers, understands that." Deston made a connection about this with several friends who retired from the Navy ("navy nukes" he calls them) who used to work aboard surface ships and nuclear submarines. For six to eight years, "they had to sit in an eight-foot-by-four-foot box that was underneath the waterline for twelve hours a day, five days a week. And their bodies were screaming at them: 'I got to go do something!'" Deston explained. "When they got out of the Navy, the last thing they wanted to do is sit in a cubicle. Half the guys I know who used to be navy nukes became tree planters making a fraction the money and benefits that they used to make—and 1/100 of the money they could make if they went back and stared at dials in the private sector. They wanted to be outside. So this whole engagement with the environment is one of the benefits."

For Deston, the team-building aspect of permaculture and small-scale, intensive farming is also critical. Conventional, fossil-fuel driven farming, he explained, can be very isolating. "You have your combine. You have your radio blaring in it. It's an air-conditioned little box, and you're driving across the wheat or the soy field, and you've got to do 400 acres between 8 AM and 6 PM." Deston compared this to farming at a small scale, which typically involves working in teams and relying on more traditional methods of physical labor. And many veterans, Deston believes, benefit from being part of such a team. "As much as any of us might feel disparaging of a chain of command, we're also going to look at our team and understand the value of the team. So individual body-mind balance and community support are two great benefits that come out of small-scale farming."

⊕ ⊕ ⊕

Many veterans are reluctant to use power tools and large machinery, and this is part of what attracts them to small-scale farming. Deston understands their reluctance. "The smells and the sounds, the vibration, the amount of noise. I definitely went through a phase where I wanted to do everything with hand tools, and it had a lot to do with the noise," he told me. "But now I've gotten to a place in my life where I've worked through all that. I'm happy to run my chainsaw," he chuckled. Then reflecting further, he added, "It actually took me 15 years to say, OK, I really want a chainsaw so that I can do this work. But I had to learn a lot about forestry and ecology because I was also scared of having a tool that was so powerful that I could unthinkingly do damage. And that was a big barrier to getting the chainsaw or doing my first project with an excavator. I didn't want to have more power than I could skillfully wield because I knew that I had a potential for doing more damage than I did good if I did things unskillfully."

These days, Deston describes himself as "a little bit more liberal" with his use of tools than some veterans. "I don't have a problem bringing in an excavator to do a couple of days of work to alter a landscape in a way that is going to halt erosion or allow for better capture of water in a keyline system. Judicious use of these tools can produce drastic, radical and quick benefits." A good example, Deston explained, is the Nisqually Delta Restoration project in Washington State, at the southern end of Puget Sound, which was the largest tidal marsh restoration project in the Pacific Northwest.[2] At one time, industrial farmers had created diversion ditches to drain the delta, so that the adjacent lands were dry enough to farm. During the restoration project, Deston described how heavy machinery was used "to recreate the meander of the Nisqually River, and to bring in large woody debris from Fort Lewis." The area also has one of the strongest returning fisheries in the region, he explained. "So the lessons that we learn from ecology are important. We can use these large tools with prudence. We can use fossil fuel to rebuild the damage that has been created through the injudicious use of fossil fuel."

At the same time, Deston sees merit in "stepping back and asking, what used to be done? And how will we do it when fossil fuels run out?" In many ways, he explained, this is the benefit of small-scale, sustainable agriculture projects. In "small-scale, high-intensity farming, you're close to your neighbor rather than being on 600 acres," he said. "So the question of fossil fuels being eliminated, making small-scale gardens, it also leads to this neighborliness, that you're working with a community or a team."

☙ ☙ ☙

When I asked about the major challenges of getting veterans involved in sustainable agriculture, Deston's answer was simple: "Congress." He elaborated, "The interest of the veteran is there, the interest of the community is there, the knowledge in the local foodsheds about how to make these changes exists. We have the human power, we have the knowledge, we have the direction. We simply lack the support of the infrastructure of political will."

Deston continued, "There are lots of veterans that are at least peripherally interested. I know dozens of veterans, right in my own area, that are very interested, if not already invested, in going this direction. And yet when we put a bill in front of Congress and the Senate and we say we want to put veterans back to work, two things happen: the first thing is that sustainable farming doesn't get written into the proposed laws. This blew my mind, completely blew my mind! The Veterans' Retraining Assistance Program (VRAP) will train bankers and real estate agents and construction workers, all three of them industries that have flat-lined or crashed, but it will not train an organic farmer, which is an industry that has shown 6,000% growth in the last 20 years. It is the only farming sector where wages are rising. And the VRAP will not fund training it. So this is a big problem."

Through the G.I. Bill, post-9/11 veterans can access sustainable agriculture training if they attend an accredited university that teaches it, Deston clarified. "But the VRAP and Veterans Vocational Rehab Training don't, and we've got a lot of veterans out here who are in the 36 and over age bracket, who served maybe 15 years ago for 2–3 years, that are now unemployed. They're qualified for those programs, but those programs don't cover sustainable agriculture training. These are veterans who may own their own house and could, on 7–8,000 square feet, feed themselves off of that property and save $7–8,000 a year, which might be enough to keep them in the house if it gets challenged for payment because they're unemployed. And yet we don't teach this program that could actually be instrumental in keeping them in their homes. This is extremely problematic."

Deston continued, "The other layer of that is that Congress didn't pass the *Veterans Jobs Corps Act*! Excuse me?" he exclaimed, his disbelief clear. This act was proposed to increase the training and hiring of veterans, with a particular focus on conservation work and maintaining public lands. "So even if we can get those programs lined up, we still don't have anything that says, 'Hey, we're actually going to support these 800,000 unemployed, perfectly able-bodied vets by putting together programs that get them out into the field, get them landed and get them jobs.'"

What struck me as Deston spoke about the different programs is that much of the work and retraining veterans are being encouraged to pursue are completely opposite the very physical, active work of being a soldier. These jobs do not provide the whole-body engagement he described earlier. When I asked if my interpretation was correct, Deston agreed. "Yeah, they're not providing that kind of engagement." For example, he added, "They're moving veterans to HVAC [heating, ventilation and air conditioning] modeling and design. So you're sitting on a CAD [computer-aided design] machine, and you design a more efficient HVAC that's run on coal," Deston chuckled. "Here's this guy sitting in this little cubicle designing his HVAC system for a 30-storey high-rise, and the HVAC itself that he's designing is going to be run by coal, so the net product of this is an unhealthy environment, an unhealthy person and a power grid that will still need updating as soon as the fuel runs out. And that's what we're investing in. It's an issue of Congressional will."

🍂 🍂 🍂

Currently, there are almost 1 million unemployed veterans and 2.2 million farms (nearly the lowest number of farms in US history).[3] "We're in a place in our society, at this time, we have perhaps 800,000 able-bodied unemployed veterans." When Deston first realized this, along with the fact that the homeless population is overrepresented by veterans, he remembers thinking, "Wait a minute! That's all solutions waiting to happen!" Through VETS_CAFE, he connects veterans and farming while also providing exposure to civilian life, since successfully transitioning from soldier to civilian requires positive contact with the civilian world. "You're still a soldier if you don't become a civilian," Deston explained.

"Our goal is to make sure there's no dysfunctional vet," added Deston. "My hope is that we're in a position where veterans who lack stability in their lives, we can begin with a mutual aid program. Now you get a little bit of stability. The veteran's no longer homeless. They have an address. They know that they're going to eat. They've got a place to do their laundry. Now they can pursue going through this grinder that is the VA claims process. But their basic needs are met."

Deston emphasized the importance of creating community amongst veterans in order to support them, and so that they might, in turn, support others. "I think a lot of veterans are a lot more willing to step out of their comfort zones or into new experiences and try things because they have been set on a seeker's path," he told me. "And that happens because stability is taken from them and resilience isn't." Accordingly, something Deston believes is most important in turning veterans' lives around is reestablishing a sense of stability, which he asserted can happen through small-scale farming. Thus, the motto he now lives by, and the words he shares with others are: "We all we got. We're going to take care of each other because we all we got."

The notion of mutual aid networks for veterans is not new. Indeed, Deston likened VETS_CAFE and similar groups popping up throughout North America to the mutual aid Bonus Army marches on Washington, D.C. in the early 1930s. As he described it, the veterans who marched on Washington during the Great Depression were saying, "Hey, look, we did our time in service. Congress made promises to us about the way it would take care of us, and that never happened. We want our benefits now."

Deston sees the 1930s marches as a useful model for veterans today. And while there are differing notions about how mutual aid support networks should operate, he explained, it is not about charity. "What we need right now is a large-scale drive that comes from the ground up, from veterans saying 'Hey, we're going to support our local food security. We're going to try to stabilize our local ecologies. And we're going to do it in a manner that our needs get taken care of.' And that might not always be a career or salaried job, but at least people don't have to live on the streets and they get fed. And we're missing on both those accounts all over the place right now."

Through its courses, VETS_CAFE intends to reach out to all veterans, no matter their generation. "I want to serve all vets," said Deston, who aims to create intergenerational dialogue between Vietnam-era, Korean-era and peace-time veterans from the Cold War era, as well as post-9/11 veterans. In addition, it's also important to reach out to the "allies" of veterans, those "who may not be veterans themselves or may not be a veteran's spouse, but who are interested in the topics that we're talking about and understand that while we're certainly focusing some portions of the program on dealing with opportunities for veterans, it is not meant to exclude."

Furthermore, while VETS_CAFE doesn't offer counseling or therapy, "we have a partnership with a State agency that does have access to those resources," Deston explained. If a veteran enrolled in a class is wrestling with something, be it an inability to sleep, not liking the pills he was given or finally feeling ready to begin a VA claim, "then we have a team waiting in the wings to get them connected to those resources and to follow through on meeting those needs. Even though that's not part of the deliverables for the class, it's part of the support for the class."

Deston also wants to find ways to form alliances with civilian groups across the US. "I think that anywhere you go across the nation, you ask the simple question, 'Hey, do you see a problem with the disproportionate number of returning veterans in our unemployment lines?' Everybody's going to say, 'Yeah, of course that's a problem.' But we all live in our own little bubble. How do we join up so that we actually can become effective in that?" he asked. "And everywhere you go, you ask the question, 'Are there as many outdoor recreational opportunities as there were 30 years ago that feel safe to you? Would you still swim in that river? Is the hike over this mountain pass still as pretty now that that clearcut's taken place? What do you think about the way these roads have been widened and we've lost all those street trees?' And everybody's going to say, 'Yeah.' But everywhere you go, people are going to have different rationalizations for why it needed to occur or different solutions for dealing with it, because they're all really living in their local bubbles. And I don't know what the answer to getting a greater momentum together is," he said and then laughed. "I'm looking for opportunities to join bubbles!"

Postscript

When I spoke with Deston in September 2013, he was unsure about the future of VETS_CAFE. He still wants to work with veterans, but for the time being, has stepped back to focus on building his permaculture consulting business, Abundance Consulting, and is producing batches of custom seedballs for conservation, agriculture and forestry projects through both non-profit and government agencies.[4] At the time of our conversation, he had just received his first contracts. "That's pretty exciting for me," he said.

In the future, if he continues his veterans work, Deston sees a need to be connected with and supported by a larger funding organization, something that is not always compatible with the independence and flexibility available to a small program. "I am interested in working with a group where we can have a small group's vision rather than meeting the needs of a large organization halfway across the country," he explained. But he's not ruling out future VETS_CAFE programs, and told me, "If I get an invite that looks any good, of course I'd do it again."

Learning to Trust Again

Steve Critchley, Jim Marland and Can Praxis

During his 28-year career in the Canadian Forces, Steve Critchley taught many soldiers how to "be army." Unfortunately, he said, "there are no programs that teach the guys not to be army." In response, Steve cofounded the Can Praxis equine therapy program with Jim Marland, a registered psychologist and Equine-Assisted Learning facilitator. Through Can Praxis, Steve and Jim incorporate horses' natural instincts to read body language to support veterans with PTSD in rebuilding their family relationships.[1]

🍂 🍂 🍂

For many veterans suffering from operational stress injury (OSI) or post-traumatic stress, connecting with other people is difficult due to the symptoms of their injury, including anger, lost self-confidence, lack of trust, a sense that nobody understands what they've been through and a tendency to disengage and isolate themselves from others, as well as to self-medicate with drugs and/or alcohol. Most families suffer along with the veteran, and repairing damaged relationships with partners and children can be difficult.

The main purpose of the Can Praxis equine program is to support veterans as they begin to rebuild their family relationships, stated Steve Critchley, a 28-year Canadian Forces veteran and one of the program's founders. In the case of a plant that has lost leaves, regrowing those leaves requires "the correct environment and the right nutrients," Steve explained. And for veterans and their families working to reconnect, "that correct environment is communication, the nutrients are their words. Being able to understand what it's like to connect with a horse helps them make the connection on how to approach people."

Most veterans who spend time on the ranch northeast of Rocky Mountain House, Alberta, gain self-confidence when they realize a horse will trust them, which then lends to reconnecting with their families. Steve explained that through interacting with horses, veterans can learn how "to change their behaviors in a way that allows the family to learn to trust them all over again." Indeed, according to Jim Marland, psychologist, Equine-Assisted Learning[2] facilitator and Can Praxis cofounder, working with a horse can be a very simple but profound experience, when veterans and their partners "realize that the horse is throwing out metaphorical, teachable moments about who they are, and how they are—in a sense representing other people in their lives." The experience that many veterans have—"when I calm down, the horse calms down"—is often easier to accept "and learn from because a horse is teaching them," Jim told me. He encourages participants to talk continuously around the animals, both as a basic safety measure (to let the horse know where they are) and as a metaphor. "If you're talking to the horse, it knows where you're at just by the volume," he explained. "But if you're sharing your heart with your spouse, your spouse will know where you're at, too."

The purpose behind Equine-Assisted Learning, Jim explained, is to use "the natural instincts of the horse to read body language." This is because in the wild, horses are "animals of prey, and they want to know if any animal—horse or cougar or human being—that's approaching them is a friend or a foe. If it's a friend, they can relax. And if it's a foe, they'd better be on their way. And they bring that ability from the wild into the domestic setting and are very, very good at reading our body language."

Furthermore, horses "crave social interaction," Steve told me. And like people, they have a chain of command, with a leader and followers. At the same time, because horses are prey animals, they "are hypervigilant all the time, even when they're relaxing," Steve said. "Individuals with PTSD/OSI are in the same sort of situation; the difference here is

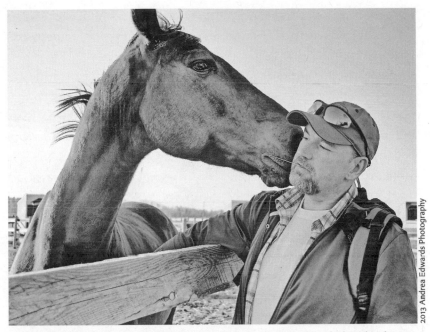

2013 Andrea Edwards Photography

Ryan Edwards, a veteran who served in Bosnia in 1999, bonded with a horse at Can Praxis. His wife Andrea said of the program, "Finding hope when you feel so lost can be a real awakening for your soul."

that it's easier for a horse to learn to trust than it is for an individual who is suffering the devastating effects of PTSD or OSI." A main benefit of veterans working with horses, Steve told me, is that they can "regain a connection with another social animal in a way that helps build self-confidence and helps bring them out of depression."

❧ ❧ ❧

"I've always been around horses," Steve explained, as he told me about the time when, at age 18 and serving in the Canadian Reserves in Egypt, he and his friends rented horses at the pyramids and ran away from their guides. He and his wife now live north of Calgary, where they breed Canadian Horses,[3] and name their foals after fallen soldiers from the Lord Strathcona's Horse (Royal Canadians) Armoured Regiment based in Edmonton. Being a horse owner for the past seven years, Steve is deeply aware of the ways that spending time with a horse can have a profoundly calming influence. "When I'm not doing well, my wife says, 'Go see your horse,'" Steve said to me, and for him, extending that influence to other veterans—and particularly those suffering from OSI—was an obvious next step.

Steve Critchley has a deep understanding of the military worldview, and "why military guys see the world black and white, right and wrong, now and then, and do something, do something!" During his 28 years in the Canadian Forces, Steve was an instructor on many leadership courses, including basic training, the Master Corporal's course, the Sergeant's course, the Warrant's course and Officer's training; he was also a Tactics and Unit Demolitions instructor.

Steve developed his understanding of the ways that trauma and mental health issues can play into soldiers' and their families' lives during his last few years in the Canadian Forces in his role as a mediator and harassment investigator. Closer to home, his daughter, a current member of the Reserves who was on the Canadian close-out tour in Afghanistan, was recently diagnosed with OSI, giving Steve an intimate and personal connection to the need to support veterans' transition to civilian life, and especially those suffering from post-traumatic stress. Over time, Steve has observed that spending time with his daughter and horses together in a therapeutic relationship has "had a very definite positive effect on our relationship," and this personal experience has affirmed that he is on the right track with Can Praxis.

After leaving the Canadian Forces ten years ago, Steve transferred his military mediation skills to "civvy street." As part of the transition, he became licensed to teach the Managing Differences course, developed by Dr. Dan Dana at the Mediation Training Institute International in Kansas City. The course focuses on conflict management through learning to navigate stressful conversations with effective communications. For a time, much of Steve's mediation work was at the international level; today, however, his main focus is disputes within Canada.

In 2010, Steve began to think about developing an equine program for veterans and how this might be combined with his mediation and conflict resolution training. He was introduced by a friend to Jim Marland, who lives on a ranch northeast of Rocky Mountain House. In contrast with Steve's long career in the Canadian military, Jim has worked for many years as a psychologist, including in the prison system, prior to which he spent a number of years working in adventure education in the United Kingdom, including teaching rock climbing, sailing, kayaking, mountaineering and survival skills.

Soon after their first meeting, a new, if somewhat unlikely, partnership emerged: a collaboration between Steve's teaching and training in Managing Differences and Jim's training as an Equine-Assisted Learning facilitator. "Jim's a different character than I am," Steve readily admitted. "He's got a different demeanor, different understanding, different way of dealing with things." And it is because of their differences, Steve believes, that their partnership works so well. "I'm there for the conflict, Jim's there for the crisis." Each brought his individual expertise and understanding to developing what would eventually become Can Praxis—"Can" for both Canada and a can-do attitude and "Praxis" for the way theory is put into practice. But it still took nearly three years for Can Praxis to become a full-fledged program, piloting its work with Canadian Forces veterans.

"The purpose behind Can Praxis is to help veterans with PTSD establish constructive communications with the person closest to them—generally their spouse," Steve told me, although that person might also be another family member, partner or same-sex partner. "Doctors, psychologists, therapists, facilitators all claim they know what's best for the individual, when in reality the person who knows that veteran best is their spouse. If individuals are able to find one safe place for a conversation, that's generally with their spouse." However, because post-traumatic stress can filter out self-awareness, conversations with partners and close family members do not always provide safety, but instead, can spiral into emotionally or even physically destructive conversations. Interacting with horses can bring awareness to the non-verbal aspects of a conversation, Steve explained, including "body language, attitude, tone, inflection." But Steve and Jim are both clear that Can Praxis is not offering treatment for post-traumatic stress; rather, it's an opportunity for veterans to work with horses to bring an awareness of self, and develop a deep comprehension of all verbal and non-verbal aspects that go into having an honest, non-threatening, non-confrontational conversation. "The concept, quite simply, is that if you can learn to communicate effectively, despite PTSD, with one person, that's Ground Zero," said Steve. "That gives you the strength, the confidence and the ability to then try it with another person."

⊕ ⊕ ⊕

After their first meeting, Steve and Jim spent the next two and a half years trying to launch Can Praxis. They knocked on doors at the Canadian Armed Forces, the Department of National Defense and Veterans Affairs Canada and were surprised and frustrated by the response. "All of them quoted the exact same verbiage as a party line," Steve told me, citing directly from an e-mail he received from then-Veterans Affairs Minister Steven Blaney:[4]

"No proof animals help people."

Eventually, toward the end of 2012, with the help of the Lieutenant-Governor of Alberta, the Honourable Don Ethell, Steve and Jim made inroads into Veterans Affairs Canada. Lt.-Gov. Ethell, who had served as a Colonel in the Canadian Armed Forces for many years, has himself been diagnosed with PTSD and is a passionate supporter of veterans' issues. Through Lt.-Gov. Ethell's contacts, Steve and Jim started months of talks with Veterans Affairs Canada, and in May 2013, Can Praxis was awarded $25,000 to conduct a study "on the relationship between horses, veterans and PTSD." With this funding and the help of University of Saskatchewan researcher, Dr. Randy Duncan, Can Praxis is contributing to knowledge and understanding about the benefits of veterans working with horses.

Around the same time, Steve's daughter created a Facebook page and Twitter account for Can Praxis. And not long after joining social media, Steve received a call from Wayne Johnston, the founder of Wounded Warriors Canada: "The first thing [Wayne] said is, 'How much money do you want?'" Wounded Warriors Canada, which later committed to sponsoring further phases of the program, was excited about Can Praxis. The organization's Executive Director, Scott Maxwell, told me that "the issue of mental health, post-traumatic stress disorder and injury generally as a result of service—it doesn't stop at the soldier. The family plays an instrumental part in that, and we hear that all the time." So when Wounded Warriors Canada learned about Can Praxis's focus on veterans and their families, Scott said, "the bulb lit, and we just thought this one seems to fit with our ideals and what we wanted to do with equine therapy."[5]

Wounded Warriors Canada provided the funding for the first three pilot programs, and with the research money from Veterans Affairs Canada, Can Praxis was able to run monthly programs from early spring to early fall of 2013. When I asked Steve about the $25,000 of research funding from Veterans Affairs Canada, which does not seem like a lot of money since Can Praxis programs are free of charge to veterans and their partners (including flights and accommodations), he confirmed that he and Jim are currently donating their time and effort. "Everything goes toward ensuring that we can run the program at no cost—or at extreme minimal cost—to a veteran and their spouse." For the moment, Steve and Jim's focus is gathering evidence that the program works. "No one's making a dime off this program or getting any compensation until we've proved that it actually works. Then we can look at how we compensate for time spent. Because generally, for the three days' work that we do, it's a minimum of five days work," explained Steve. "That doesn't keep the mortgage people happy."

⊕ ⊕ ⊕

Set on Jim's ranch, nestled into the quiet countryside outside of Rocky Mountain House, Can Praxis offers a three-phased program. Qualifying is simple: "If you're a veteran with PTSD, you just qualified," Steve told me.

Phase One offers three-day programs that concentrate on establishing the safety of having a conversation with a partner, spouse or close family member. Each Phase One program runs with a maximum of six couples at a time. It's important to keep things small, said Steve, both "so that people are a little more comfortable, and so they can't hide in the wallpaper. They have to be part of the thing. And we do push them out of their comfort zone."

The first day at the arena is open to the veterans only. Jim meets with the veterans' partners in the boardroom of their hotel to listen to their concerns, their experiences and their hopes. The partners then have the remainder of the day to themselves; some choose to do local sightseeing together, while others rest in their hotel rooms. With the veterans, Steve and Jim start with classroom work on theory about conflict and communication, followed by groundwork with the horses (no riding happens in Phase One). The horse work involves various activities ranging from taking the horses for a walk to specific exercises in individuals and pairs, which Jim explained, "are low-level obstacle courses where people go around barrels and over poles and do problem-solving exercises that demand effective communication."

The purpose of working with only the veterans for the first day is that "we need the guys just to operate and relax and get to know each other and feel comfortable, and not have spouses looking over their shoulder," Steve said, noting that his use of the word "guys" is non-gender specific; although, since the Canadian Forces comprises 85% men, the majority of veterans are male. This initial period creates an opportunity for the veterans to connect with others with a similar background, despite their different Army, Navy or Air Force trades. "In this program, they share a common bond, and it's a real strong one," Steve told me. "It doesn't matter what trades they used to be, what components, what elements (Regular Force, Reserve), how old they are; none of that matters. That first day and a half is pretty powerful for them to reconnect." The partners then join the veterans, and receive the same theory lessons and instruction with horses.

A central aspect of the Can Praxis program, Steve explained, involves teaching specific conversation skills. "We're focusing on conversation, on communication, so that the spouses and the veterans can find a way that works for them—it may not work for any other couple, but who cares?" he said. "If it works for them, that's all that counts." Steve finds it helpful to use military terminology when working with the veterans, such as "'IAs [immediate actions] and stoppages,' or 'IAs and secondary drills.' Those words define things we train guys to do immediately when something happens," he explained. "When the feces hits the rotating oscillator, you've gotta do something, do it now." Steve applied the concept of immediate action to conversations between veterans and their partners, and particularly to conversations that have the potential to become emotionally or physically destructive when a veteran is experiencing a crisis moment. "We're teaching the veterans and/or the spouse to have a code word that they share," Steve explained, "And if either or both use this code word, the immediate action is to stop the conversation and back away."

Steve drew a parallel between this code word and a minefield drill: "You hit a minefield, you stop. It's the first thing you do," he said. "Then you retrace your steps out of it to a safe place. Same thing for having a conversation that's gone sideways and is now becoming destructive. First step is: stop the conversation." However, the secondary action, or what happens next, is also crucial, since the code word is only a temporary stop, not an avoidance technique. Accordingly, Steve explained, the secondary action involves "how to reenter that conversation. Even if the conversation started about butterflies, something happened that caused it to go sideways, so the conversation needs to be finished. To finish it, you need to approach it in an appropriate manner at the appropriate time. That's where the theory and the interaction with the horses come in: to help them see what they need to do to enter into a conversation so that it's non-threatening and non-confrontational."

🍃 🍃 🍃

Because Equine-Assisted Learning relies on horses' natural instincts, the horses are not trained specifically for therapy work. "I can't train those instincts into a horse, they've got them already," said Jim. "You can't even take them out of the horse—not that I'd want to." The majority of the horses involved in Phase One are Haflingers, which were originally bred in the Austrian village of Hafling to be workhorses. Many traditional religious communities in North America, such as the Hutterites and Mennonites, continue to use them for farm work, but Haflingers are now bred for various other purposes, from dressage and trail riding to general leisure activities. For a time, Jim and his wife bred Haflingers, and while they no longer do so, they currently have 15 horses, most of which, Jim said, "are fairly calm, easy-going horses." For each program, he brings in horses with a range of sensitivities and personalities to work with the veterans and their partners. "I might select one or two that are really bomb-proof, and one or two that are a bit more sensitive."

Jim further described the benefits of working with a horse: "The participants and Steve and I get to look carefully at what the horse is doing. And if the horse is relaxed and following, chances are that things are all well with the person on the exercise. But when the horse stops, starts swishing its tail or disregards the person altogether and just walks away, that's a signal to everybody that it's good to ask a question." At that point, or when the exercise is finished, Jim might say, "Look, old Sid was following you quite easily until you got to the barrel and then he wouldn't move. What was happening?" The observation, followed by a short open-ended question, he explained, gives the participants a chance to describe what was happening—and that it was something noticed by the horse. "The horse is a great teacher. He'll let you know when something's not quite right or when it is great, so I follow the horse's lead," Jim said. "Oftentimes, it's much easier for the veterans to talk

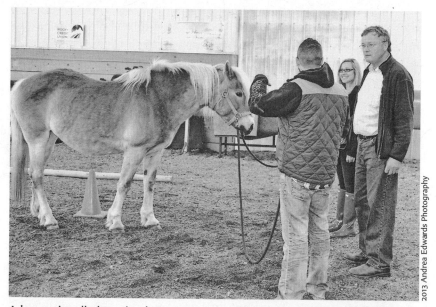

A horse signalled tension between Aaron and Shannon. They used skills to resolve it while Can Praxis psychologist Jim Marland looked on.

about it when it's been pointed out by a horse, than some psychologist who asks the difficult question."

Jim takes Can Praxis participants through a range of activities with the horses that require them to use their communication skills and body language to lead a horse through a particular activity—often without touching the horse. And as they work with different horses, "we talk about the horse's personality, how sensitive it is, how obedient or how willing—and oftentimes spontaneous metaphors about human relationships spring out of those experiences." In fact, as the veterans begin to transfer their learnings from the horse to their human relationships, very often they will say, "You know what? That horse is behaving just like my son," Jim told me. "And they know exactly what they mean—I might not—but they see similarities between the horse's behavior and someone else's behavior, and this observation often results in profound insight and a change in the way they understand a situation."

Jim remembered a spontaneous moment on one program when he took veterans and their horses for a short walk through the bush. "They loved that," he recalled, and they asked if they could to it again, this time on their own. "The sun came out and it stopped raining and we had half an hour to spare, so off they went, just to be alone with a horse in the bush. For most people, that was something they'd never done before." The exercise is not an official Equine-Assisted Learning exercise, but because of the intensity of the program, it gave the participants "a chance to be quiet and reflect," explained Jim. Chores and cleaning the stables are also built into the program, he said, to "lower the level of intensity so that when it gets intense again, they can take it in."

When I ask Jim more about how veterans benefit from working with horses, he explained that it is because the "horse oftentimes replicates people in their lives. The horse responds to the veteran in a way that people respond to the veteran. For example, the horse might get upset, maybe because the veteran is very stressed," said Jim. "And then another veteran will work with the same horse, and that horse will be quite calm. So the veterans learn greater and deeper self-awareness about how they're relating to other people and about how other people—their spouses and kids—relate to them."

Once the veterans and their partners complete Phase One, they become members of a closed-group, alumni Facebook page. "We want these guys to help each other," Steve told me. "And we don't want to become the crutch. Jim and I want to work ourselves out of a job." However, Can Praxis also plans to bring the veterans and their partners back for Phase Two. This phase is still conceptual, but the plan involves another three-day program during which veterans learn to care for and ride horses. Evenings will be spent reconnecting with the learnings from Phase One, "having conversations about what's working for them, and what they need to work on." Steve and Jim intend to run several Phase Twos for veterans only, and at least one for partners only. Bringing back the veterans and partners separately will allow them "to reconnect with people in the same situation," while at the same time allowing Steve and Jim "to measure and understand where they are with the learnings from the first phase and any fine-tuning required."

This phase will be followed by Phase Three, a three- or four-night pack ride in the mountains. "And once again it's bringing the guys together so that they have an opportunity to reconnect and network, and to see where they're at and help them fine-tune their ability to communicate," Steve explained. In order to go on this pack ride, the veterans will need to demonstrate the "ability to deal with some stresses and be able to communicate effectively through them. And not everyone will want to do it. So it's those who want to and those who demonstrate that they would be the right fit at the right time."

While much of Phase One takes place in a more constructed environment—a barn—Phases Two and Three will be outdoors. Learning to ride the horses will happen outside, and the three- to four-day trail ride in the mountains will, Jim hopes, provide veterans with an ability to "reflect on their lives from a distance, [with] a new perspective."

In addition to planning Phases Two and Three, Steve is working to find other locations throughout Canada where it might be suitable to run Phases One and Two. It's expensive to bring veterans and their spouses from across Canada to small-town Alberta, and it would be more efficient for Steve and Jim to travel to various locations throughout the country. For consistency and standardization, the cofounders would always teach and run Phase One. However, if they are able to find and certify several locations across the country, it might be possible to run Phases Two and Three out of these locations. In addition, the purpose of certifying other ranches is that if Can Praxis participants want to continue spending time with horses, they would have a safe space to do so that is closer to home. According to Steve, "What we need to do is ensure the facility, the people, the horses—all of it—is appropriate. We'd have to have the right atmosphere, it would have to be a positive location that promotes the same values and ethics that we have, the first one being, of course, no harm to people—or to animals."

As with many other programs for veterans, Can Praxis continues to face challenges. Getting participants is a major one. Many veterans sign up, only to cancel at the last minute. "Twice as many people refuse at the last minute as people who show up, which is to be expected with the group we're working with," Steve observed. This is compounded by the fact that, for some reason, "3rd Canadian Division, the Canadian Armed Forces' Health Services, are not playing nice." They have told people to stay away from Can Praxis, despite the fact that soldiers from other parts of the country are getting leave passes from their Commanding Officers to take part. "We've had units within 3rd Canadian Division try to send people, and they've been stopped," Steve added, his frustration and disbelief clear.

Jim suggested that the business side of things is also difficult, particularly when marketing their program to people who haven't thought much about the intrinsic and intuitive connections between humans and nature and the ways that horses can be a profound way of intervening in veterans' lives. Despite "generations and generations of anecdotal data offered up by people who know horses," said Jim, "our major challenge is selling it to bureaucrats who represent large organizations who need ample data before they can spend a dime." Accordingly, Steve and Jim are hopeful that their research partnership with the University of Saskatchewan will provide empirical data to support their program.

Steve and Jim are realistic in their goals and know that Can Praxis's program is not going to work for everyone. One question that arises is, as Jim put it, "to what extent is it a lasting change?" And the reality is, despite society's yearning for a method that will fit all cases, "there is no magic solution, there is no magic bullet, there is no one-size-fits-all," Steve conceded. "What we're doing is providing opportunities for veterans to leave with real, practical take-away skills, and then it's up to them to use [those skills]. And to do that, we sometimes have to push people out of their comfort zone."

A story that will be familiar for many veterans suffering from OSI is that, for some veterans who arrive in Rocky Mountain House, their comfort zone is their basement. "We've had people on the program that won't talk to other people, or who hide all day in their house with their curtains closed," Steve explained. Those veterans' comfort zones had become, more or less, nonexistent. Accordingly, he and Jim understand part of their work as helping the veterans to expand their comfort zones. "When they show up the first morning, [some] have extreme states of anxiety," Steve recalled. "And by the time they leave, they're laughing, giggling and having a good time."

Where each veteran is along his or her journey through post-traumatic stress and recovery when they come to the program also plays a role in the extent to which their experience with Can Praxis will manifest in lasting change. "Most of us find change difficult," said Jim. "We're asking these guys to change a huge amount: dropping their guard, trusting other people, having a positive outlook, thinking that they'll live longer, not having to be fearful all the time. Those are big challenges." Jim speculated that while most of the veterans get "enough salutary experience to promote long-lasting change" during their time on Phase One, the extent of the change will depend on how the veteran is able to engage in the lessons offered by the horses, and by Steve and Jim.

Both men are adamant about the fact that Can Praxis's focus is always the present moment. "We don't dig into the traumatic event; we don't even go there at all," Jim explained. "We don't dwell on the past," Steve added. "It's important for the people we work with to understand quite simply that the past exists. The past carries emotion. And it's important to acknowledge that emotion from the past, but be focused on the present. In other words, for lack of a better term, 'where the fuck are your boots right now?'" Occasionally, the past does come up, and when that happens, Steve said, "We attend to it, and we move people to the present. And with that, once people become focused on where they're at now, it's what do you want to do about it tomorrow. And then how do you communicate that?"

An additional component in working toward lasting change involves teaching veterans and their partners to "look for a small success, every day for the rest of their lives." Steve went on, "The idea behind success is that you and your spouse are satisfied, whatever that looks like; satisfied doesn't mean you're happy, satisfied means you're in a better place than you were before. It's not about chasing rainbows or unicorns, it's about what is a realistic moment that causes satisfaction. It's to focus on that so that it becomes a way of life, so that you're not thinking about it anymore." By way of example, Steve offered an analogy to which most people can relate: "Remember the first time you went to drive a car? There was a lot to learn, and it felt uncomfortable? You don't even think about that stuff when you jump in the car anymore."

If the veterans gain one thing from their time in Rocky Mountain House, Steve hopes it's "the confidence and ability to have one successful conversation a day" with their partner. Because once they gain that confidence and ability, it eventually becomes easier to talk with someone else. But he was also realistic: "There's always backsliding, and that's part of what the alumni Facebook page is for—to actively encourage them to have conversations amongst themselves to attend to that stuff."

Steve also made clear that Can Praxis is not providing marriage counseling. "If it turns out that the best thing for them to do is separate, then that's the best thing for them to do. We're not going to create artificial expectations." At the same time, Steve believes that many of the spouses find his own military background helpful because he helps them to understand the veteran's military worldview, behaviors and seeing things in "the stark realities of this or that." Part of Can Praxis's goal is to support veterans in seeing the world as civilians do, "not in black and white but in color." One particular exercise that helps with this,

Steve added, is Join Up, in which the participant is in a round pen with a horse. "You have a whip or a horse stick with a plastic bag attached to it, and you just rattle that thing around and wave it. This causes the horse to run away from you," Steve described. "What we're demonstrating is that's your family running away from you every time you walk into the room. That's the kids running and hiding for cover, the wife looking for an excuse to leave the house, because your attitude—everything that you bring into the house—*you* think you're cool, calm and collected, but in reality you're everything but. You think you're being assertive when you're actually being aggressive."

In the round pen, "when you act like that, that horse runs away from you in fear," Steve explained. "But when you drop the stick and adopt a physically relaxed attitude, that horse will come over to you and actually nudge you after it decides you're no longer a threat. So what we're showing is that yes, you may have done damage to your family, but if you adopt the correct behaviors, then your family can come back to you and learn to trust you all over again. And so it can be pretty powerful when guys make the connection—and spouses as well."

"Each Year I Feel Better"

Christopher Brown and Growing Veterans

When Chris Brown left the US Marines at 22, he struggled to reintegrate into civilian life. Eventually, on the advice of a counselor, he started a small garden box on his apartment balcony. Today, in addition to tending a raised garden bed in his backyard, Chris runs Growing Veterans, a project to get more veterans involved in farming and to establish a network of small-scale farms that will hire veterans and support their transition to civilian life. Chris believes that "Being able to grow food, bring life back into the world and sustain life, is a huge factor when it comes to guys with this type of background."[1]

🌿 🌿 🌿

It was through advice from his counselor that Chris Brown started a small one-foot-by-two-foot garden box on his apartment balcony. "It was a difficult transition for me," Chris told me, recalling his posttraumatic struggles and difficulties reintegrating into civilian life in Whatcom County, in northern Washington State. After leaving the military, he recalled, "I was coming from combat and feeling isolated; there weren't a whole lot of people around that really understood what I had been through." A Purple Heart recipient for injuries received during the suicide bombing of his patrol base, Chris served three tours—two in Iraq and one in Afghanistan. Forty-one Marines from his unit were killed in action during those three deployments, and Chris has confessed that he senses he could have been one of them.[2]

Thinking back to that transition time, Chris told me, "My counselor kept giving me ideas of things I might do to reconnect with myself and where I'm at with home." Eventually, the counselor suggested that Chris try growing a plant, and Chris decided to grow something practical—that is, something he could eat. "I'm of the mindset that if what you're growing can't be used for food, then I'd rather spend my time growing something that can." But by his own admission, that first foray into gardening wasn't particularly successful. Chris attempted to grow four different plants in one hanger box on his balcony, but none of the plants grew very well because "there wasn't any space for them to grow, for their roots to set." One of the plants Chris grew was mint, which is invasive and often takes over other plants growing in its vicinity; this is what happened in his hanger box. "The mint's roots took over everything else and strangled them. I thought that all plants would grow harmoniously and that it would be a lot easier than it actually was, but just through that observation I was able to see that there's a lot of complexity that goes into growing food—or plants in general—and in a lot of ways, gardening reflects the complexity that we deal with as people."

Even though the mint overtook the hanger box, Chris recalled with fondness the time he spent watering and caring for his small garden, trying to keep the plants alive. "I started to learn what plants need to thrive, and part of that is more space, more sunlight and different types of nutrients. And learning these things gave me a new hobby; instead of thinking the intrusive thoughts that guys like me can have, I was spending more time thinking about growing food and how I could improve the garden for next year." As he worked over the summer to keep his garden alive, Chris and his wife drank tea daily from the fresh mint leaves. "My wife and I thought that was really cool, to be able to take something that we grew and use it for something that we could consume to help us either stay healthy or just enjoy a cup of tea. I guess that little hanging box is when I first started to think about growing food differently."

When he was young, Chris's family occasionally had a garden, "but it was never an instrumental part of my life," he said. Today, Chris thinks differently and speaks fondly of the five-by-twelve-foot raised garden bed he built in his backyard. "That's about all I have room for," Chris admitted. "But now my garden is to the point where we can go out and harvest stuff for dinner. This season, we had beets, onions, snap peas, tomatoes, garlic, spinach and chives—a wide array of things we could use each night for dinner.

"And being able to grow food—to pull it out of the dirt and an hour later be eating it for dinner whenever you want—mentally, it's awesome, and physically it helps my body to stay healthy because if you've got a healthy body, you've got a healthy mind. And also the physical activity of preparing the dirt, preparing the plants, preparing the plot.... There are so many things that [gardening] helps: mental, physical, emotional, spiritual. Growing food, if you're conscious of what you're doing, there are a lot of different pluses." Chris laughed.

Most important, perhaps, was Chris's realization that, "Each year the garden's gotten better. I've been able to produce more food out of it. And each year I've been feeling better as far as my PTSD symptoms go, too. For somebody who has been around death and bad things, to bring life back into this world is a really therapeutic thing. And also being able to bring that food to someone else to sustain their life is doubly important."

🌿 🌿 🌿

Chris joined the US Marines right out of high school. Both his father and grandfather had served in the Navy, and his step-grandfather was in the Army in Vietnam. "That had a small influence on why I joined," Chris recalled. More significant in his decision were his feelings of indifference toward high school and his lack of interest in pursuing further education. Also important, he said, "I saw what the folks who stayed around town were doing with their lives, and I didn't really want to stick around and have that happen with me."

But perhaps most important of all, Chris was drawn to the sense of adventure and excitement advertised by military recruiters. "I wanted, as they say, to 'test my mettle,' and see if I could hack it; to see what I was made of. I wanted to experience what the military was like, and part of me wanted to see what war was all about. I was pretty naive at the time, but I guess I got all those things," Chris admitted. "I always tell people that when it comes to my military experience, I wouldn't change it for the world, but I also wouldn't wish it upon my worst enemy because

I learned a lot of good things but a lot of bad things had to happen to learn those lessons."

In addition to nurturing plants and a garden, Chris has also found relief through contact with other veterans. As he struggled to readjust to civilian life, he observed, "The more I got involved with local veterans' groups, I realized that there's some therapeutic value in just being around other vets."

While attending Western Washington University, Chris wrote several papers about veterans' transition to civilian life; these captured the attention of one of the leaders of Vet Corps, a local veterans' group monitored by the Washington State VA. Vet Corps works with veterans transitioning to civilian life to help them obtain higher education and navigate the veterans' system through representatives at colleges and universities across the state. After meeting with Vet Corps officials, Chris was offered a position as the first Vet Corps representative at Western Washington University. As part of his job, Chris was sent on a trip to Israel, accompanied by three other student veterans, where they spent a week with wounded Israeli veterans and experienced a peer-to-peer support program the Israelis had created. When the four Americans returned home, they turned to one another and said, "We need to start something like this."

Together with a few other friends, the four veterans set about creating a pilot project to emulate the Israeli peer-to-peer support program. This involved monthly weekend retreats for young veterans, so that they could just spend time together, sharing stories and camaraderie. However, Chris recalled, "We weren't having the level of success that we were expecting," pointing to differences in both culture and geographic size between the US and Israel, which Chris believes made it difficult to imitate what the Israelis were doing. "In their culture, they're more open with their feelings; it's a lot harder to get American military combat folks to share what's going on with them." However, Chris doesn't consider that the project was a complete failure because he learned a lot from the experience. Since then, the group has had some growing pains, and some of the original members left while others joined. Chris himself left, since the group is in Seattle and he and his wife live in Whatcom

County, but he remains on the organization's board, as he put it, "trying to help them keep going and keep the mission alive."

Instead, as Chris worked toward completing his bachelor's degree in human services with a psychology minor, he began to contemplate further what he jokingly called the "side effects," or the positive residual effects, of peer-to-peer support and working the land. As he explained, "I just started to tie all this together, and I knew that I wanted to start something that tied in veterans, sustainable agriculture and the broader community." In a series of fortunate events, Chris was approached by a Korean War veteran, with a similar vision of training veterans in small-scale agriculture, which helped Chris begin to solidify his plans.

"There are a lot of veterans' groups out there, and a lot of them bring veterans together to hang out with each other, which is good—but vets are still isolated or not recognized by the broader community," said Chris. "And when you're trying to transition home, that's an important piece that's missing." While still in university, Chris met regularly with a small group of other veterans to brainstorm what such an organization would look like. However, by the time they graduated in June 2012, they still did not have anything firmly established, so many of the others moved on to other jobs. Chris, however, continued to be taken with the vision. "I really saw a lot of value in it, and I found a way to work on it."

He obtained a six-month community service fellowship through The Mission Continues, which provides post-9/11 veterans with fellowships to serve with non-profit organizations in their communities. Chris's partner organization for the fellowship was Growing Washington, a non-profit that focuses on sustainable agriculture and improving economic and social health in Washington State. Chris's mission was to develop Growing Veterans, a project to get more veterans involved in farming. As the organization's Director, Chris saw Growing Veterans as providing an opportunity for veterans to work in sustainable agriculture while also connecting with one another and the wider community. The group's mission statement became "to foster an environment where military veterans are empowered to be responsible stewards, leaders, and active participants in their community—and to share the lessons we've learned about humanity with the world."[3]

As part of the fellowship agreement, from August 2012 to January 2013, Chris split his workweek. He worked part-time (Tuesday through Thursday) on Growing Washington's Community-Supported Agriculture (CSA) program, a job completely separate from Growing Veterans. Then Friday through Monday, Chris volunteered his time to create Growing Veterans. Growing Washington did not pay him for this work, but for the fellowship period, he received a monthly cost-of-living stipend from The Mission Continues.

Chris's fellowship paid off, and Growing Veterans became operational in the spring of 2013. While not all his original plans have come to fruition, Chris is proud of how far the organization has come. "Most non-profits take three to five years to get operational," Chris told me. "This is our first year, and we're already producing crops and having all sorts of volunteers and projects going." Chris is mindful of all the help and support the organization has received, as well as a number of fortuitous events and people who have come into his life.

In spring 2013, a three-acre parcel of land, previously used by the Bellingham Food Bank, came up for lease. The landowners wanted the property to continue to be used by a non-profit charitable organization to grow food, and with the help of Growing Washington, Growing Veterans took over the lease. "It's a great fit, and we were really lucky to get it," Chris observed. There are two greenhouses, in which they are currently growing tomatoes, and a shed with a tractor that Growing Veterans can use. The land also came with several rows of raspberry bushes that the veterans harvested in late June and early July. While they needed to set up some irrigation and a few other aspects essential to running the farm, the fact that Growing Veterans took over a space with most of the necessary amenities enabled them to hit the ground running.

Another aspect crucial to Growing Veterans's success is the continued support of Growing Washington. The two groups are currently piloting a relationship in which all food grown and harvested by Growing Veterans is distributed through Growing Washington's CSA program. In exchange, Growing Washington pays the lease on the land, the utilities and Growing Veterans' staffing costs. At this point, it's not clear whether the relationship will be financially sustainable, but Chris was optimis-

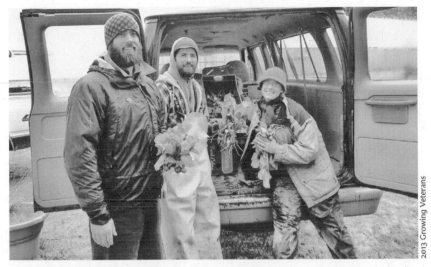

The early season crew sends off some early Easter Egg radishes grown in the greenhouse; Chris Brown stands center.

tic. While he admitted that they might not reach the break-even point in 2013, he suspected that they would do so in 2014. "We've learned a lot this year already about what we could do differently to create higher-value crops and help us be sustainable," Chris observed. In addition, to generate funds, Growing Veterans had several fundraising campaigns planned for the fall and winter months, and Chris was hopeful that with that, Growing Washington would want to continue the relationship into the next year. "If not, we'll adjust our focus and keep going," Chris suggested.

✤ ✤ ✤

As Director of Growing Veterans, Chris had grand ideas at first, but in a lesson valuable to many start-ups, scaled back his plans when he realized the importance of building a base of support, "both through getting veterans involved and through networking with other local agencies and other local farmers." In addition to growing food, Growing Veterans is working to establish a network of small-scale farms that will hire veterans. "We want to act as the go-between for all things veteran and all things sustainable agriculture," Chris explained. "If a veteran comes to us wanting to be involved, depending on what they're doing, where they are in life—if they're looking for a job, or if they're in school and want an internship or if they just want to volunteer—we'd like to be able to turn to the network of farmers and farm agencies and tell them, we have a veteran who's looking for this, can any of you provide it? Or if they have job openings or volunteer project requests, they can come to us and then we can go to our network of veterans' groups and do the same thing." In particular, Chris and his team are focusing on local and regional food systems. "There are a lot of flaws with large-scale, monoculture-type agriculture, so I think having veterans support local sustainable food systems might give it more respect from people who might not otherwise pay attention to it."

Currently, about ten veterans come out to the Growing Veterans farm at least once a week. While a few of them come on a strictly volunteer basis, Chris does everything he can to help veterans get paid for their work if they express a desire to become more involved. Some of the veterans have obtained an internship through the G.I. Bill, which provides education benefits to post-9/11 veterans. Through this, veterans get paid and earn college credits while working on the farm. In addition, Growing Veterans hosts several fellows through The Mission Continues. And alongside Chris's own job as Director, Growing Veterans provides part-time employment for another veteran. Meanwhile, Growing Washington has hired two additional veterans to work within their organization, one of whom comes out to help on the farm once a week. Starting in September 2013, Growing Veterans also had a full-time staff member, through Vet Corps, to "help build up our network of military bases and veteran agencies as well as be a resource referral person for veterans who are working out at the farm."

As Chris explained, "we do all these as professional development for veterans because a big issue for veterans is unemployment and the difficulty translating skills they gained in the military onto their resume to gain civilian employment. And so we try to create opportunities to get veterans involved so that they have something for their resume that's in the civilian sector, something that uses the skills they gained in the military and that, in theory, will help them secure employment down the road. Or help them get into a good college."

Another important focus for Chris is developing Growing Veterans' website, which he sees as essential to reaching out to both veterans and civilians. The site features a blog section called *The Horn*, where veterans are invited to submit their stories as "a way to bridge the gap of understanding between the general public and the veteran population." A Growing Veterans staff member works with the veterans to refine their submission as necessary, and then it is posted to *The Horn*.[4]

The website also features Op Wire, which is intended to connect veterans with jobs, internships and volunteer opportunities in sustainable agriculture, particularly farm work—or opportunities with an agency or educational program that supports sustainable agriculture.[5] Since Op Wire was launched in June 2013, when many farmers had already done their hiring for the season, Chris has worked on making farmers and different agencies aware of it; he is hopeful that its success will grow. Indeed, while Growing Veterans tends to be local and regional in focus, Chris sees the website as an element that can serve veterans across the country. "I'm hoping it will attract a lot of different folks who wouldn't normally be exposed to issues related to veterans or even issues related to sustainability or sustainable agriculture. And I hope that having these things on our website will bring people to it and that they'll learn more about us and then want to support us through donations or connect us to a resource that we're not aware of."

Chris is the first to admit that he owes part of Growing Veterans' success to his full-time farm manager, who before joining Growing Veterans managed the Food Bank farm on the same property. While not a veteran, "in her previous life she was a mental health counselor, so she's a pretty good asset to have out here because she already knows the land," said Chris. "And she knows how to talk to people who've been through trauma, and she's been through trauma in her own life as a civilian. So I don't think any veteran out here is bitter at the fact that she's not a vet; she's a really good person and has helped the farm do well." In particular, the farm manager keeps the farm's day-to-day operations running smoothly, which enables Chris to work in the office, both building the website and networking with other farms and agencies. "It's been really nice having that, because if I had to worry about all the crops and everything, I don't think we would be developing nearly as quickly as we are," Chris admitted. And when he does come out to the farm, about four or five days a week, Chris acts primarily as another farmhand. "My farm manager and I work together on the planning for our crops, but for regular day-to-day operations, I leave everything up to her and I just come and say, what needs to be done? And we make it happen."

As mentioned in several other chapters in this book, some veterans with post-traumatic stress are triggered by the sound and/or smell of power tools and avoid using them for this reason. Chris, however, is not affected by the noise or smell, and he noted that while it might be ideal to rely mostly on hand tools for veteran-run farms, "it's not very practical unless you have a lot of people involved. When it comes to using tractors, I think that it's really hard to measure whether or not it's valuable. It would be really cool to get some draft horses or something like that to till the land, but even that takes a lot of work, and also a lot of knowledge that I don't have," Chris admitted. "I guess the line I cross is when it comes to chemicals and things like that. I have no interest in using chemicals to help grow crops. I prefer using natural plant species that attract pests instead of spraying all these crazy chemicals, which in turn make the food less healthy. But when it comes to just using a tractor to weed or to plant, I don't see a huge deal with that."

🌱 🌱 🌱

The biggest challenge, Chris has found, is that "there's not a whole lot of money" in farming. He told me, "We need to find a way for veterans and farmers to get paid more because the bottom line is that the work that they do is absolutely necessary for everyone. And it's a shame that they don't make very much money doing it." Growing Veterans' current fiscal sponsorship through Growing Washington has alleviated some day-to-day worries about money and paying staff, at least for the year when Chris and I spoke; however, Chris worries constantly about finding ways to raise money and break even so that Growing Veterans can continue its relationship with Growing Washington into the future. In addition, he said, "a lot of the vets who get involved here have great ideas that we could use to continue developing, but we don't have any money to fund those ideas."

Awareness is another challenge for Growing Veterans, both on the veteran side and the civilian side. "If a veteran isn't aware that there are opportunities in farming, they're not going to go for them. So that's one of challenges we face as we move forward: to find ways to make veterans aware of what we're trying to do and to find ways to sell the idea as one that can be of great value." As part of coping with this challenge, Chris continues to work on building connections in town as well as building a relationship with a sustainable agriculture training program that is scheduled to start at several local colleges near Seattle in the next few years.

Another aspect of this challenge lies in helping civilians become aware "not just of veterans and farming but of veterans in general," Chris told me. "Post-9/11 veterans come from the past ten years of war, trying to rebuild nations, working diplomatically with local community leaders, busting our butts 24/7, for 7 months on end. We know how to work hard, and we have a lot of soft skills like leadership, teamwork and decisiveness under stress; those are the three big ones that help veterans, especially in farming. But having the community aware that veterans have these skills and showing them how they can tap into it...if the community is aware, there's going to be much more recognition for the veterans that are in the community, and it's going to help address again some of those multifaceted problems, like homelessness and unemployment."

Chris also echoed the sense of being misunderstood that I've heard articulated by many other veterans. "Some community members that I talk to completely respect and acknowledge all that veterans go through," he said. "But others see a veteran as a symbol of destructive militarism and all this crazy stuff you see on the news." In reality, Chris continued, "most veterans got out of the military for a reason. Some folks got out because they didn't like the things that were going on in the military, and if they are interacting with a community member who views them as that symbol, it can be really destructive in the way that they interact with each other. I think that's why a lot of veterans isolate themselves, because of that misunderstanding."

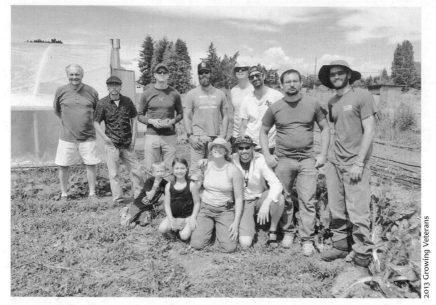

Some members of Growing Veterans on a summer Friday harvest day with Chris Brown right.

Toward the end of one conversation, Chris shared a different and more positive kind of memory from his time in the Marines, when he spent much of his time in rural areas living amongst the local population. When out on patrol or working amongst locals in Iraq and Afghanistan, Chris saw how people were living: "They make do with what they have. They built their homes out of earthen mixtures, and they farm the land that they are living on," he reflected. "And seeing that lifestyle made me think about the way that we live our lives over here, and these people—besides the fact that they had troops living where they were trying to raise their families—for all intents and purposes, they were pretty happy. And I think that probably had an influence on me when I got back here, thinking back on those times and the lifestyle that they had. I wouldn't necessarily want that lifestyle, but being connected to your food and the people you live with and next to is something that's positive that I think would help us out over here if more people were focused on it."

Accordingly, Chris argued that gardening and farming hold "a lot of therapeutic value for guys who've been around death and destruction and bad things." An added benefit of small-scale community farming is the ways it can help veterans transition to civilian life: "When it comes to veterans transitioning right now, they have higher rates of suicide, higher rates of mental health issues, homelessness and unemployment. And what I'm trying to do is address all of those. And so when it comes to farming, not only does it address the mental health stuff, but it also addresses employment, which also can address homelessness."

In this, as Chris continues to work toward his own healing, he described his primary mission as Director of Growing Veterans: "I just have to keep being persistent and find ways so veterans can keep working out here on the farm and being able to support their families at the same time. I think that's probably my number one concern: being able to keep vets here and also let them be able to live their lives off the farm at the same time."

Moreover, Chris told me, "when you consider that in the US, within the next 10 to 15 years, the majority of current farmers are going to be retiring, there's a big niche there that veterans can fill. And I think that getting veterans into that role as helping to take over sustainable agriculture or agriculture in general if they don't really care about some of the values behind sustainability—regardless it's helping to get veterans jobs, and it's using veterans to help improve their communities by bringing in food. So it's a holistic response to a lot of problems that returning veterans face."

A Chance to Prove Myself Again

Gordon Cousins

✤ ✤ ✤

While training to become a Canadian peacekeeper in Vietnam, Gordon Cousins was injured and nearly died. In the years after the accident, he was often overcome by sudden angry outbursts and difficulty sleeping. While never diagnosed, Gord suspects in hindsight that he suffered from post-traumatic stress. In 1997, Gord reenlisted in the Reserves and found that his new role gave him focus. He was also spending more time outdoors. Based on his own experiences, Gord emphasized the ways that human experience in the outdoors takes on a different rhythm that contrasts sharply with the demands of modern urban life.[1]

✤ ✤ ✤

The first time I met Capt (Ret'd) Gordon Cousins, C.D., as I extended my right hand to shake his, I was struck by momentary paralysis and unsure what to do. Gord, a tall slim man in his mid-60s with short greying hair and a friendly smile, chuckled kindly. It was not the first time in the last 40-some years he'd been greeted by this reaction. He gently guided my right hand to meet his, showing me that we can still shake hands, despite the fact that he's missing all five fingers.

Unlike many of the other veterans I've interviewed, Gord did not grow up with plans for a military career. Rather, he joined the Lorne Scots regiment of the Canadian Forces' Reserve Army after a falling-out with his Boy Scouts' troop leader. Gord had been active in the Scouts until age 14, but after leaving the organization, he wasn't sure what to do with himself. Then, in 1963 when he was 15, Gord met some other teens who were parading with the Lorne Scots, and he told his father, "I'd like to go, too." So the two of them went together to explore more carefully the commitments involved in joining the Lorne Scots. Because of his experience as a naval officer during World War II, Gord's father was initially not keen on Gord joining the Canadian Forces. However, his father eventually consented and enlisted him, since it would keep Gord him away from the television and off the streets. Unlike his father's own war experience, being in the Forces also did not seem particularly dangerous since his son would not be going overseas.

His father's conviction to keep his son out of combat was made clear a few years later. When Gord was 17, his father was offered a promotion and an opportunity to move to Camden, New Jersey, to become the head of engineering for the Campbell Soup Company. But the move was unthinkable. The Vietnam War had just started, and with two teenage boys, his father declined the promotion because his sons would have been drafted into the US Army. While he considered taking the job and leaving the boys to live with their uncle, in the end Gord's father decided it was more important to stay together as a family. "I was well aware of the impact [that decision] had on my dad," Gord said. "It was the end of his career. He never got promoted again."

So Gord continued serving as a part-time soldier with the Lorne Scots while he finished high school, and over time he described, "It grew on me." However, his father's conviction that his son would not be going overseas when he enlisted was proven wrong. Gord volunteered for the extra training required to become a peacekeeper in Vietnam. Then, on May 7, 1968 at the age of 19, Gord was injured when a booby trap simulator blew up during one of those extra training sessions. He lost all the fingers on his right hand and severely damaged the hearing in his right ear. A 21-inch-long piece of shrapnel pierced his right collar bone in two places, opened the top of his right lung and stopped within a ¼ inch of his spine. During surgery, when the doctors removed the shrapnel, they couldn't stop the bleeding and Gord went into cardiac arrest, nearly dying before doctors were able to restart his heart with adrenalin.

Gord spent the next 15 months recovering in and out of hospital, including one period of 6 months in a row, during which time he suffered from staph infections, shingles, pain and nausea among other symptoms. Gord described all of these experiences as "one form of stress that builds." In 1971, once he was considered to be "patched up," Gord was discharged from the Reserves with the status "Struck Off Strength" (SOS) and received a financial settlement to compensate for his injuries.

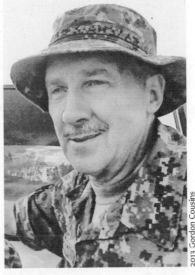

Gordon Cousins

2013 Gordon Cousins

In addition to his physical injuries, Gord now suspects that he also suffered from post-traumatic stress as a result of the accident. If he was driving down the street in a friend's car and another car backfired, Gord would immediately duck below the window. He also remembered standing in line when someone nearby stomped on a paper cup, which caused him to wince and duck. During the years following the accident, Gord often woke up, tense and sweating, from nightmares in which he was "approaching some catastrophe but not going through with it. Or committing some gross thing," he said. "I can remember in the immediate post-op period, vivid and morbid situations of me garrotting people, running people over with a vehicle, sliding off a roof and not being able to hang on because of no fingers on my right hand."

Gord also recalled his tremendous anger, and what he refers to as "a killer instinct coming out," despite never having been on the front lines of combat. In the years after his accident, Gord often threw things out of frustration. The army had designed a number of prostheses for him, including special pens, eating utensil holders and "carry systems," but he soon stopped using them because he was too frustrated. "I decided that I would start the journey of doing without the stuff. And I guess in hindsight that helped, but there were frustrating times and embarrassing times."

Gord had many clumsy and awkward moments in those early years. "I'd be out on a date with a girlfriend and I'd be cutting my steak, and the methodology was such that it would sometimes slip and so my peas would go on the next table and maybe a few minutes later the potatoes would go in the opposite direction." He remembered feeling both embarrassed and frustrated while he excused himself to clean up the mess. And overall, he described how this period when he was learning to do everything with his left hand caused "a build up of anxiety—or anger would probably be more accurate...I didn't take the anger out on other people as much as it was a stress-reliever for me—but it hurt people or bothered people when they saw it happen."

⊕ ⊕ ⊕

In 1967, the year prior to his accident, Gord had spent the summer working in the Parc national de la Gaspésie, a national park in the Gaspé region of Québec. "I was out pretty much by myself on Montagne Jacques Cartier," Gord explained. "I did prospecting there, and I found a gold mine." Gord was looking forward to continuing this work the next summer, and one of the first things that flashed through his mind after the accident was that he had messed up his summer job. "I felt really bad because, as a student and a Reservist, every summer I was going out to the bush, and I wasn't going to be able to go. That was a major thing that flashed through my mind: 'I screwed up my summer!' And I knew it instantaneously because I could just see the tendons dangling there on my hand."

Gord's boss came to visit him in the hospital, told him to concentrate on getting better and that he could always return to work in the bush the following summer. As it turned out, in the summer of 1969, his former boss arranged for Gord to be hired as part of a geophysical exploration team with another company based out of Thompson, Manitoba. Gord was discharged from the Canadian Forces' Barriefield Hospital in Kingston, Ontario, and a few days later, he arrived in Thompson. "I had this sudden transformation from parading every morning in gray flannels and a white shirt at the foot of my hospital bed for the Matron to inspect," he explained, "to three or four days later being in Thompson, Manitoba."

As the logistics coordinator for a team of field workers collecting soil and mineral samples, Gord ensured that the team received all necessary field supplies, and he then repackaged all their samples to be shipped back to Toronto. "Because I had been in hospital and I was in poor shape physically and I was skitterish, gun-shy, underweight et cetera, I didn't have to live out there but I chartered aircraft, and I flew out there," he told me. Gord believes the job was an essential part of his recovery. "That immersion really rapidly put things behind me, and I felt useful. I felt I was engaged. It was the beginning of a feeling that I really had a role to play. I was able to get back into shape during the three months I was able to work before I went off to university."

After spending the summer of 1970 as a cross-cultural exchange student in Ghana, in 1971 Gord returned to work for his former boss from 1967. "He took me to the Ungava Region in northern Québec, and then in 1972, I went to the Albany River district flowing into Hudson's Bay," he said. "We canoed and we flew by helicopter, and we would set up a wall tent and stay in this location for three weeks and then we would move to another location and do some more stuff. We were constantly outdoors. And other than the fact that I would cut my hand and snag it on trees and I couldn't feel it and blood would flow, I had a great time. And nothing held me back; so that was a therapeutic experience—it just erased pretty well all the skitterishness I had about having been hurt."

After completing his degree at Brock University, Gord moved west to Calgary, where he boarded with his aunt and uncle. During the winters, he often took solo trips out to the Rocky Mountains. "I would snowshoe in, pitch a tent, stay for the weekend, maybe do some target practice with my .22, and then I would hike out and get back in the car and come back to Calgary." In the summers, Gord regularly snorkeled in the mountain rivers, "just free flow, like a tourist, looking and fetching whatever I found on the bottom."

"And so I would stay close to nature in those areas," he recalled. "I found it relaxing and rewarding. It was an environment where there was no lid on the pot, so there was no pressure buildup and it was easy to do what I wanted when I wanted to for those short stints of time."

At the time, Gord didn't make a connection between nature and his recovery from physical and psychological trauma. It is only more recently that he's begun to wonder whether his recovery and adaptability are associated with all the time he spent outdoors. Nature, he said, "gave me a chance to prove myself again. And I didn't really dwell on it very much other than the fact that I was looking to soak up every new experience I could to adapt," he explained. "I had no counseling. I didn't have any understanding of what could happen. So at that point, I was more personally proving myself, just like an educational program, as opposed to anything therapeutic. But it's only in retrospect now that I feel I reintegrated pretty well because of that."

Gord credits both the Boy Scouts and the Reserves with his love for nature. Reflecting on his decision to enlist in the Reserves once he'd left the Scouts, Gord knew that he wanted to be outdoors. "I felt more comfortable in the big outdoors than I did confined—the concept of being confined in a ship or in a plane above ground with gravity issues bugged me. So I thought of that as the happy medium," he said. "I continued aspects of the outdoors all those years. That's one commonality that continued before, through and after my rehabilitation time. And I feel that I accommodated myself to my situation better because of it."

Recovery, however, is rarely a straightforward process, as Gord explained. "You make much progress forward, then something happens and you're three paces back." In the 1980s, with the busyness of working and raising a young family, Gord got away from his active outdoor lifestyle and experienced what he calls "throwbacks to that anger thing." He recalled times when if touched by one of his four small children while he was asleep, he struck out automatically at the child and was then horrified by what he'd done. Other times his anger would suddenly boil over while he was in the living room, and he would put his coffee cup in the kitchen sink ten feet away by throwing it like a grenade. "I didn't raise my voice, didn't hit my wife, but that was an expression of built-up frustration. No more cup, followed by tears, embarrassment," he said, then paused. "I don't do that now." Gord also recalled slamming doors, and told me how "one time my son didn't hear me speak, and I bashed down the door to his bedroom. I felt like a heel afterwards, yay tall," Gord said, showing a one-inch space between his left index finger and thumb. "He's crying, I'm embarrassed, and so on. And so those were some things that I've pretty much overcome."

In the early 1990s, the movie *Legends of the Fall* was being filmed in the foothills west of Calgary. When the producers put out a call for extras with previous military experience, Gord volunteered as an amputee. However, he quickly found that his work on the film was triggering his previous traumatic experiences. "I'd come home in the morning after filming all night, and I'd close my eyes and this flash would go off between my eyeballs. I started to react in ways I had not for years," he admitted. "I would wake up suddenly in a 'panic state.' Now, that's not serious—but it was interesting how something like explosions on a movie set triggered these flashbacks and these thoughts. Stuff returns with simple, stupid little things," he explained. And then reflecting on the ways that his personal experience might apply to other veterans, Gord said, "I think there can be a recidivism rate that needs to be understood and not frowned upon. There shouldn't be a lot of sanction brought against a person who is recovering over various lengths of time."

When I asked Gord how he overcame his anger and outwardly antagonistic reactions, he told me that even though filming *Legends of the Fall* triggered his traumatic experiences, the film also rekindled his love for the outdoors. In 1994, Gord signed his sons up for Cadets and became a parent volunteer. He saw the Cadets as creating a positive environment for his sons, where they would learn important skills such as time management, prioritizing and developing focus—skills Gord believes they carry with them to this day. His volunteering also led him to spend more time outdoors again.

For the first few years, no one with the Cadets asked Gord about his missing fingers. Then, late one evening, the Commanding Officer (CO) of the Calgary Highlanders Army Cadets Corps came out to Gord's bivouac site under a pine tree and sat down. He said, "Cousins, you know something about this stuff. What did you do before?" After hearing about Gord's experience with the Lorne Scots, the CO asked him to reenlist. Gord recalled being surprised. Since the Canadian Forces' policy to that point had been, as Gord described it, "If you were hurt, you were out," he thought the CO was teasing him. "I thought and assumed that they wouldn't take somebody with 'missing parts.'" However, the CO's request was serious, and Gord, feeling proud and happy to be allowed back in to his previous family, reenlisted in the Reserves in early 1997.

Gord found that his new role in the Reserves gave him "something to focus upon. I was able to go out in the bush more and more," he said. "I did like all the exercise. And we did some creative stuff. And so that was a very good replacement." He also started snorkeling and playing underwater hockey again, among other activities. "I found that I was now once again useful, and so I think 'the military' helped in having a role," Gord explained. "It helped stem a lot of that issue: abruptness, sudden anger, sudden outbursts. I didn't wake up in the night. I slept right through. Little things like that."

Gord was the first amputee to ever take a canoe course with the Canadian Forces, and some of the course instructors were surprised to see him there. He recalled how he was clumsy with some of the strokes, but he persevered to become competent in a canoe once more. "If I didn't master it the first time, then I would say, 'I didn't do that right. I want to do it again.' And the instructors said, 'OK, what didn't you do right?' 'Oh, this, this and this.' And they would allow me to redo it, and I eventually mastered it to their standard," Gord recalled. "And that was a further confidence builder. It made me feel useful, and I was fulfilling a practical task that they wanted. I still do it."

For many years, in addition to running his own small business, Gord was a Logistics Officer with the Cadet Instructors Cadre and an Instructor in Canoeing and Swift Water Rescue with the Cadet Corps' regional expedition center in Calgary. When needed, he also trained Cadets in Calgary and the surrounding region in skills such as bushcraft, navigation and cold weather survival. Each summer, he went up to the Yukon for three weeks for the Cadets' Long Paddle, which Gord described as "therapeutic but in a different way. I get out of the desk, I get paid to be outside, having a 1,000-kilometre canoe trip that's good for the soul.

But it's not because I need it therapeutic wise; it's because I enjoy it. I'm putting something into the kids, and I get paid to do it."

In August 2013, after spending eight weeks at the Whitehorse Cadet Summer Training Centre in the Yukon and leading his last Long Paddle expedition, Gord reached the compulsory retirement age of 65, with a total of 22 years of service in the Reserves. When we last spoke, Gord was uncertain about what his future would hold. He planned to continue running his small business and hoped to remain attached in a civilian capacity to the Cadet Corps' regional expedition center, perhaps doing weekend training work with Cadets. "I do always think 'What am I going to do now? Do I go out and buy a canoe to get outside?'" he asked. "I'd like to maintain that connection with the outdoors now that I'm retired. And I have a torn heart because I have little kids that I should teach—in my own family, my grandkids—and then there are the older ones that I could teach, too, as a civilian instructor. I just need some time to decide."

When I asked about the outdoors and what nature means to him, Gord thought for a moment and then said, "The outdoors, regardless of what you do—you climb, canoe, hike, those types of semi-physical activities—it's something that places you in control of your own self. You're not encapsulated in the city. You're not having a general routine. You're not doing predictable, repetitive things, and you have to use some of your wits and some of your personal skill set. And so it has the ability to quickly separate you from things, the stress of the city, accommodating your life to either your circumstance or your community. You're out and away. And it doesn't matter whether it's winter or summer, I think it's that separation that allows you to have a measure of control over your own life again. That's how I can articulate it," he said, then went on. "You just feel more fulfilled, in control. You're more aware of the things around you rather than having to respond to every circumstance."

Toward the end of one conversation, Gord expanded on his thinking. "I like the free flow environment of being out in the bush, doing something I'm familiar with. There's a certain tempo and schedule. There are always exceptions and something suddenly might change, but it's not something that's beyond your ability to control," he reflected.

"When you're out you just go by the rhythm of the outdoors, of the soil, of the season. Day turns to night, you stop. Light comes in the morning, you get up. There's a rhythm that's much different than somebody yelling at you to do this or that, or you having to punch a clock at a certain time."

"Life Is Good Now"

Shepherd Bliss and Kokopelli Farm

Born into a long-time military family, Shepherd Bliss was raised to be a warrior, but resigned his commission before going to Vietnam. He suffers from sound trauma due to various experiences during his military upbringing, his own military service and his later time in Chile. While in his early 40s, Shepherd bought a small farm and credits farming as one of the most beneficial activities in managing his trauma experiences. In January 2013, he adopted a Catahoula leopard hound named Winnie, who has brought many joys and is enabling Shepherd to make deeper relations with people than ever before.[1]

⚜ ⚜ ⚜

It was a midsummer morning when I first talked with Shepherd Bliss, a US Army veteran, part-time college professor and owner and operator of Kokopelli Farm in Sebastopol, Sonoma County, Northern California. His gentle, peaceful voice described the view from his window. "I'm looking out on beautiful trees now. They're waving at me...their partner the wind comes along. We're here in the Redwood Empire. Life is good. It hasn't always been that way."

Now in his late 60s, Shepherd told me about his life. "Demilitarizing myself has been 40-some years. I was militarized the first 20, 25." The first of five children, he was born Walter Shepherd Bliss III at the end of World War II into a military family. (Fort Bliss, the US Army post in Texas, is named after his family.) Shepherd's father, a military officer, was away at the time of his birth, and his mother was "a peasant woman from Iowa." Due to his father's military career, Shepherd and his four siblings were raised on military bases and moved on a three-year cycle.

Coming from a long line of military officers and named "Walter" after his grandfather, a naval officer, Shepherd never questioned that it was his destiny to be in the military. As the first-born, he was often called "Number One," rather than by his first name. And he admitted that he was raised to be a warrior: taught chess and military strategy at age four, often yelled at and marched around by his father. When Shepherd was old enough, he enlisted in the Army and did basic training at Fort Reilly, Kansas, which he admitted, "was actually OK for me." Elsewhere, he has said, "I did like boot camp, being with other teenage boys, playing in the woods."[2] Afterward, he began serving in the Army during the Vietnam War and had requested a post in Vietnam, which he saw as a way to move up quickly through the ranks.

All this was changed, Shepherd said, by the first woman outside his family that he "ever really loved." It was the 1960s, after he had been commissioned into the Army, and his then-girlfriend took him to a gathering at which Martin Luther King, Jr. was the keynote speaker. After hearing King speak, Shepherd underwent a radical personal change: he resigned his commission before going to Vietnam. Around that time, he also found out that his given name Walter means "warrior," and asked himself: "Do I want to be called that the rest of my life? Or could I use the name Shepherd, which is my great-great-grandmother's name?" He referred to his decisions to leave the army and to begin calling himself Shepherd as the "first major adult decisions of my life."

Leaving the military was not a popular decision with his family. "I'm kind of a black sheep," Shepherd said. "When I left the military, they were not happy. I basically resigned from the military and the family." And while he has worked carefully to demilitarize himself during the past four decades, Shepherd accepts that his military upbringing will always be a part of who he is. "I honor the military virtues like discipline, organization, working in teams, country love, sense of mission. I just don't appreciate the context in which those are applied. I'm not anti-military. I think for some people it's the right thing. I honor the role of the protector and the guardian, while not agreeing with wars in Afghanistan and Iraq."

After leaving the military, Shepherd earned a doctorate from the University of Chicago Divinity School. He then spent time in Chile during Salvador Allende's democratic government. He had planned to become a citizen there until Augusto Pinochet's military coup in 1973. Shepherd had already left the country, but after the coup, his fiancée was tortured and his best friend, Frank Teruggi, was tortured and killed. Reflecting on his military upbringing, his own military service and his experiences in Chile, Shepherd shared that "there is a whole lot of conflict and trauma that comes from the military for me." For a while, he told me, he escaped into academic excellence through various academic positions, including at Harvard and New College of California. This, he confessed, "had its merits, but also when you're doing that, you're not necessarily growing emotionally." Indeed, Shepherd eventually realized that due to the traumas he suffered earlier in life, including his military upbringing and his time in Chile, he was suffering from moral injury (better known as post-traumatic stress)[3] and in particular from what he terms *sound trauma*.

In "Sound Shy," a personal essay he wrote for *Veterans of War, Veterans of Peace*, Shepherd described himself as "usually oversensitive to noise, but even more so when...under stress."[4] He also wrote:

> Much of my behavior is sound-avoidant. I often feel a misfit in our increasingly noisy society. If I go into a room with a battery-powered clock, I can hear it ticking. If someone has an old, predigital watch on their wrist and is close enough, I can hear it ticking, ticking, ticking, so methodically. I leave such loud rooms. Those ambient sounds become magnified to me; they thunder and produce headaches. And most refrigerators are too loud for me. I usually build a little room outside the house to contain the refrigerator.[5]

Shepherd revealed, too, that while he values solitude, at times he craves contact with other people and will venture off his farm into local towns.

"Sometimes the interaction with people goes smoothly. But at other times, a few sounds can touch me off, overwhelm me, and create a 'Get me home!' feeling."[6]

Shepherd does not remember much of his time in the military or his time in Chile, and he attributes this to psychic numbing. This type of memory loss can protect trauma victims, but as he explained, "sometimes, something—often a sound—triggers me. I go to an uncomfortable place. But after years of counseling, rather than a flashback or dissociation, I tend to just go cold, chilly, distant or numb. I've gotten better at managing these moments, though I try my best to avoid them."[7]

Shepherd also shared that he has difficulty remembering names, which he attributes to his time in basic training. "One of the things I remember my sergeant telling me in basic training was: 'Don't learn the first names of anybody till you've been in combat for a while, because you can't grieve being intimate with that many people.' And that's really stayed with me," Shepherd admitted. "And what it is, is a difficulty in having a long-term relationship with them because they'll die. Of course, we'll all die." Then he added, "Death feels like it's always in the room for me, and I'm past denying it."

🌿 🌿 🌿

While in his early 40s and living in Berkeley, California, Shepherd began yearning for something different. He found himself reminiscing about the time spent on his Uncle Dale and Aunt Elva's farm in Iowa during his youth. And he realized that this is where he had been happiest in his life, and that he "felt better with fewer people around and more plants, animals, and natural elements such as water and rocks."[8]

Shepherd has fond memories of the farm. "We used to stack the hay. We didn't have electricity," he told me. "People don't realize that in the late 1940s, early 1950s there wasn't electricity in the rural Midwest, so we had an outhouse, no running water, but an ice box, a windmill and gas lanterns. At night we had stories instead of TV. Life was good." He paused, then continued, "And just getting up while it was still dark and milking the cows and then coming back to huge pancake breakfasts and cinnamon rolls. It was a wonderful life: slow, contact with animals and plants and bees and good friends. It was different than the more violent military family into which I was raised. At the farm I got away [from my military upbringing]. It was a different scene, animals and plants and hanging out with chickens and piglets and watching their community."

But despite his fond memories of the farm, Shepherd did not set out to buy a farm and become a farmer. "Funny," he told me, "it wasn't really fully a decision, or an act of will. I thought I wanted a country home." After a full year of searching for the right place in Sonoma County, about an hour from Berkeley, Shepherd learned that a 93-year-old woman had recently died and her small piece of rural land might be for sale. "I came over here. I turned into the driveway, and I said, 'I'm home.'" The woman's son, who was living next door, told him that the family was planning to put the property up for sale in a few days. "I'll be making an offer tomorrow," Shepherd told him. His offer was accepted, and ten days later, he moved into the place he would eventually name Kokopelli Farm, after the Anasazi deity Kokopelli, a humpbacked flute player and wounded healer. In some legends, Kokopelli was also "a man of the peace," explained Shepherd, someone who was accepted wherever he went, even by warring villages. And he was a trickster, whose role was anti-authority. Accordingly Kokopelli didn't take himself too seriously: "If a spiritual process became too sacred or pious," Shepherd chuckled, "he'd lay a fart; he'd just let the gas go."

When he first moved onto the farm, Shepherd recalled, the property was a mess. "I needed to burn off a lot of prunings. I needed to fix the roof," he said. "It's a humble, simple place. It's not big. It's not elegant. It's just minimal. It's big enough for me." He decided to leave his college teaching position and become a full-time farmer (although he eventually returned to part-time teaching, most recently at the Dominican University of California). And even now, Shepherd connects his time on his Uncle Dale's farm with his current life as a farmer: "I remember enjoying playing in the dirt, mud and puddles as a boy. Farming gives me an excuse to continue such play."[9]

"The farm is a pretty safe environment," Shepherd told me when we spoke. "I don't have to deal with many people, and when I do, I'm the captain of the ship here." Indeed, while he acknowledged the helpfulness of both individual and group counseling in his life at various times, Shepherd credited farming as one of the most beneficial activities in managing his trauma experiences. The other beneficial activity is his continued participation in the Veteran Writers Group led by writer, poet and peace activist Maxine Hong Kingston. Shepherd has belonged to this group for the last 20 years.[10]

Shepherd reflected on the ways farming offers a different form of healing from conventional therapies: it is, he explained, "not a 'talking cure.' In fact, it is the very opposite: it is not-talking."[11] Indeed, some of the main benefits of farming, both for himself and other veterans, are in the ways that "it gets us away from people," Shepherd said. "You have some contact with people, but basically you have to redirect your energy to the plants and/or animals. And it's not talk therapy. It's the bees who work together, the ants who work together, the gopher snakes who eat the gophers, the badgers who make holes. In this case it's the wildlife as well as the farm life, and also in this case it's in the wetlands, it's in the uplands of a marsh, which has a rare plant. So it's the whole community of the land."

Shepherd described his first encounter with a rare lily, which he believes was the particular moment when he realized that Kokopelli Farm was helping his recovery: "We have a rare plant here that exists nowhere else in the wild, and it's protected by the federal government and the state government. It's not on my farm, but at the bottom of my farm. And I'd heard about it, but when I first saw it—it's a lily, big, and it looks like it's bowing down. And I just fell to the ground and wept when I saw it. What a treasure. There was something about the wholeness of this, about the connection of this, about everything—the sounds."

Shepherd also expressed that growing food for other people has been central in his recovery. In particular, he grows and sells organic boysenberries as his main crop, as well as blackberries and Golden Delicious and Rome Beauty apples. For a long time, he also kept free-range chickens and sold their eggs. "When I came here, the place was a mess. It had never really been farmed. It had been gardened, but the berries were not up on trellises; they were mowed every year. There was something about the recovery of the fruit that enabled my recovery. And financially, even though I charge a lot for the berries because they're very labor-intensive, I don't make a lot of money from them," he said. "[The farm] helps integrate my writing life, my physical life; it's my best health insurance. It enables me to think, have a lot of solitude, be my own boss, be independent. Military veterans like that. They like not having a boss. I mean, there are lots of differences, of course, but they like the freedom. So I like the freedom here. Nobody tells me what to do."

Sound trauma will likely always be a part of Shepherd's life journey. This is the reason he uses only hand tools, such as scythes and machetes, on his farm. And on occasion, he still finds himself triggered by the sound of power tools on adjacent properties, leading him to sometimes wonder whether he shouldn't try to find a quieter place. But from our conversation, Shepherd's love for and devotion to Kokopelli Farm is clear. When he was offered a professorship at the University of Hawaii, he did try to move away, although he did not sell his farm. Shepherd moved to Hawaii for three years, and even bought a rural place there, which he also turned into a farm that grew tropical fruit such as kava kava and noni. But he soon found himself homesick for Kokopelli Farm, and returned to California where he has been ever since.

Shepherd enjoys his life as a farmer and, for many years, his role as guardian and protector of his chickens. "I get up early every morning, before the sun, I have a good sense of time. I'm punctual. I pull weeds out of the ground even though they're anchored. I yell back at my livestock, because if you don't, they won't follow your orders. They want the freedom, I provide the structure. If they fly the coop, they stay out there and the predators will eat them. There are predators in the world. Some nation states are predatory. Some of them have drone airplanes that are predatory and kill whole villages. So one has to be a guardian and a protector. And have those different archetypes within them."

He continued, "In farming you have to protect your animals. You have to have weapons, whatever they are—pellet guns, BB guns or .22s, depending on what kind of predators you have. Here we have mountain lions, coyotes, great horned owl. Of course all of those are wonderful animals, but you have to build a structure that they can't penetrate, but then there are others, like raccoons and skunks, that it's really hard to keep out. So what is the balance? I have a scythe that I mow with and a machete, so I have weaponry. But it's by hand, it's not automatic weapons like the terrorists have. The real terrorists, all of them, on both sides."

⊕ ⊕ ⊕

Shepherd observed how during his more than 20 years of living on Kokopelli Farm, some of the personal walls he has built up around himself have gradually started to come down. "By interacting more with the plants, animals, elements, I find that I have improved my relationships with other people and with the community around me," he reflected. "My friends inform me that I have become a better person because of my work in the soil and with farm animals."[12] Elsewhere, he has written that "farming has moved energy from my brain into the rest of my body."[13]

When I asked him to expand on the ways that engaging with nature moves energy from his brain to his body, Shepherd shared some of his experiences from the Veteran Writers Group led by Maxine Hong Kingston. "One of the things that Maxine leads us in is a walking meditation. We go out, where we meet, where there's giant eucalyptus, and we walk, slowly. Now, for some of the vets, that was hard at first because they're used to walking point, which means you're in the front when you're going into the jungle looking for the so-called enemy, or you feel it in your body that you'd be the first one to be shot at. But after a while, you really get into the wonderment of knowing that you are protected and there is no threat, so you walk it out. Your body sees the land, not as a place to be scorched with napalm or that's concealing somebody who could hurt you, but it's welcoming. And so you begin to transform that."

The sensory stimulation provided by farming is also expressed through Shepherd's personal writing. He has written, "When the wind sweeps through the bamboo, it soothes me, as if it were a harp."[14] Elsewhere, he shared: "I enjoy watching and hearing chickens dance, talk to each other, clown around, dig into the Earth with glee, and herald the dawn."[15] The first time we spoke, Shepherd told me more about how much he loved watching his chickens. "Chickens have a lot to teach. They have chicken wisdom. They're also prey. They're very curious but they're flighty. They can get hurt, and everybody wants to eat them. So they have prey wisdom, which is, they're kind of batty and loony, much smarter than people think... one human on one chicken, the chicken will usually prevail unless the human has a tool."

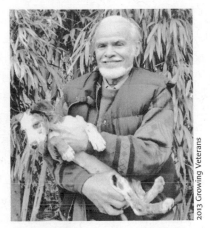

2013 Growing Veterans

Shepherd Bliss and his Catahoula leopard hound Winnie

While Shepherd used to sell a lot of eggs from his free-ranged hens, a bobcat in the area started killing them, and he gave the remaining chickens away. Instead, he turned the chicken run into a free dog park. In fact, at nearly 70 years old, Shepherd described how he became a dog owner for the first time. In January 2013, he was at the Sebastopol Farmer's Market to buy some food. "I was not looking for a dog, much less a puppy," said Shepherd. But as he was walking, a 12-week-old Catahoula leopard hound puppy named Winnie ran up to him, and when he bent down and opened his hands, she jumped right in. He looked around to figure out where she belonged and found a family with two young children—and a litter of six other dogs. Shepherd asked if he could walk around with the puppy for a while, and then did so, checking in about every 20 minutes. Three hours later, he returned for the final time, and the family told him, "She's adopted you. You should take her home." Shepherd wasn't sure, and responded, "I'm not a dog person. I don't have any space for her. I don't know what I'm doing! I can't do that." But after a few moments, he changed his mind; he decided not to think about it and just to take her home. "Of course she was not house-trained, so first she pooped in my car, then she peed in my car," he recalled. The two stopped at the pet store on the way home to buy some food, a collar and a leash. And that day, Shepherd said, with clear emotion in his voice, he realized that "something's been sent to me, and I just have to respond."

From then on, Winnie has brought much joy and many new experiences into Shepherd's life. "She's totally in present time," he reflected.

"And she doesn't remember a lot, and she's not futurizing, so it can break some of the control that the trauma has, because you have to re-orient yourself to her needs as one would to any young being in their life. And she's just there, doing what she does, without judgment, without connecting it to something that might happen, or something that did happen." And perhaps most importantly, Winnie is helping bring Shepherd into the world in new ways. "What's happening with me now is the dog's unconditional love, and my caretaking is enabling me to make deeper relations with people than I have before. There's been this block: I'll only go so far, and either find a way out or do something." In addition, Shepherd reflected, he's always preferred to spend time with a small group rather than with one person. "One-on-one has always been harder for me. That's more intimate," he said. "But with Winnie, it's almost as if there's a third presence that somehow brings a certain amount of safety."

Because of Winnie, Shepherd also finds himself meeting people with whom he would never have been in contact before. "People notice her. She's got six colors, very touchable, and a diamond on her back. She's the most incredible dog that many people have ever seen." In addition to setting up the free dog park on his farm, Shepherd takes Winnie to another local dog park from time to time. "And it's just easy, you don't even have to say much, it's kind of a dog-loving culture." He eventually hopes to train her as a service dog, but in the meantime, she works on his farm and sometimes goes with him to his college classes, where she has a calming effect on his students. Indeed, the first time he took Winnie to his speech class, Shepherd realized just how much she relieved his students' anxiety. "Winnie is a natural anxiety reliever," he commented.

When he was a young man, Shepherd decided never to have children. "I had a wonderful marriage," he said, telling how the end of his marriage came about, primarily due to this decision. "Before we got married, we agreed not to have children because I was afraid I would not be a good father. It was her second marriage, my only one. But then she got to a certain age, and she decided she did want children. So I agreed to renegotiate the contract, but I realized that I didn't trust myself. I didn't have a good model of fatherhood," Shepherd reflected. "My [other] fear was that it would be a son and that the [warrior/military] genes would prevail in spite of [my wife's] sweetness and her Buddhism, and then I'd have a killer on my hands—even if it was legal killing. I decided, 'I'm not going to perpetuate these genes.' Now, as it turns out, all the children of my brothers and sisters tend to be more like where I am—not quite in this extreme, but they're less conflictual than we were raised to be. Sometimes I think: Was it the biggest mistake of my life not to have a child? But then I think: No, I wasn't ready in my 30s and 40s, and this is fine."

Now Shepherd speaks of Winnie as "the child that I refused my wife. People in the dog world—or everybody—just call me her papa." And one of the spinoffs of owning Kokopelli Farm is that it has brought young people into Shepherd's life in a way he never thought possible. Many parents bring their children to the farm to buy berries, and the farm provides an important context for both work and play. Adopting Winnie has further enhanced the context for relationships with children. With her, Shepherd feels even more able "to relate to children, and to nurture them."

Shepherd himself had no grandfathering. He never met the grandfather after whom he is named, and his other grandfather was killed by lightning on his farm in Iowa. And yet, "all of a sudden, I've been captured by the grandfather archetype," he told me. "These toddlers just keep walking into my life. I'm being reparented by toddlers!" he laughed. Shepherd has become an honorary grandfather for a six-year-old boy whose parents bring their dog twice a week to Shepherd's dog park. And a toddler who comes regularly to the farm has announced his intentions to move in with Shepherd when he grows up. Shepherd finds great joy in these new-found relationships with children: "It's safe, intimate contact, which has been hard for me, maintaining relationships. In the military, you move every three years. So, not being on a three-year cycle is hard for me. And being in an ongoing relationship is hard for me. I would theoretically like one, and I find these appropriate women but either they or I, at a certain point, opt out."

❦ ❦ ❦

Over the years, and drawing on his own experience, Shepherd has become a strong advocate for the healing power of nature. In 2011, he became active with the Horses Building Communities program in Sonoma County, which uses equine therapy to support military men and women and their families at all stages, from pre-deployment to reintegration into civilian life. As with other groups doing such work, Shepherd said, "We had a little trouble fundraising, so we haven't been able to implement the whole program." However, through this group, he was led to SkyHorse Ranch run by Ariana Strozzi, and Shepherd told the incredible story of what happened to him there while taking part in an equine program. Each of the participants was asked to go into the round pen with a horse, and part of the exercise involved asking the horse for something they need. "Everybody was volunteering to do this but me. And I was afraid of being rejected by the horse," recalled Shepherd. "Finally Ariana said, 'Shepherd, I think it's your turn.' So I went out...it was a mare by the name of Lily. And what I wanted to work on—what I kept repeating was—'I want to work less and play more.' But after a while, Ariana interrupted me and said, 'Shepherd, you're not saying that in a very playful tone of voice,' which I didn't realize, but of course she was right. So I started saying it in a playful tone of voice. What did the horse do? Everybody who was watching this was astounded, even the horse people had never seen anything like this: the horse flipped over on her back and started throwing dirt all over herself. And what did I do? But flip over on my back and throw dirt all over myself because she was having so much fun. So she obviously understood what I was asking for, and she delivered it to me. It was a totally non-rational," he recalled. Before that, he'd had doubts about whether equine-assisted therapies really work. But now, Shepherd said, "It does work, in a very mysterious way."

While Shepherd has been spending less time with the horse community since Winnie arrived in his life, he continues to support the work of Horses Building Communities and to be involved when he can. The other important aspect of being involved with the group, Shepherd said, "is it brings me back in touch with the larger military community, not just those of us who eventually became anti-war. I find that I have things in common—that's part of finding my way back to my family and realizing the value of military virtues."

Shepherd also belongs to the Farmer Veteran Coalition, whose mandate is to create agricultural work opportunities for US veterans returning from Iraq and Afghanistan. In an article for *Countercurrents*, Shepherd reflected further on the benefits of farming:

> Sometimes dealing with people is just too much, especially when they are mean, cruel and even deadly. Times come to take it to the trees, vegetables, animals and elements. They can hold it. Weeds help me. Pulling them out can release anger—better than punching someone. Livestock appreciate attention and vigorous conversation. They bark, bellow, howl, scream and make all kinds of sounds; they listen better when one yells back, which can be a release.[16]

And Shepherd hosts others on his farm, including veterans, and provides what he calls *agro-psychology* or *agro-therapy*, which he equates with the larger green care movement in Europe.[17] "Here we hang out; we do something productive; we go for walks. We value solitude. We let people be. We get things done." And now and then, Shepherd does some informal facilitation work around the picnic table. "Sometimes the men will open up when it's not a clinical room or clinical environment. It can also happen in the clinical ways, but there's something about the healing power of the regenerative Earth, the grass, the leaves, the flowers, the bees, whatever wanders in, the ants while they're doing their work and the honeybees that don't sting."

Making a Case for
Green Care in North America

Field Exercises has chronicled stories of strength and perseverance in the face of many obstacles and sometimes great suffering. In writing out these veterans' stories, I came to hold a deep regard and affection for each of them. They generously shared aspects of their lives that many of us consider private, with the aim of supporting and providing wisdom and hope to others who have had similar experiences—and also guiding civilians to move beyond stereotypical impressions and assumptions toward a deeper and more nuanced understanding of veterans' diverse experiences.

Both the empirical research and the stories I have gathered here point overwhelmingly to the fact that when a person finds and/or remembers her/himself in ecological relationship with their surroundings, their human psyche is changed, and sometimes transformed, by the experience. Nature contact, however, is not often incorporated into conventional therapeutic and medical interventions for military personnel in North America. Indeed, in 2006 an essay in a special issue of the medical journal *The Lancet* noted that "in the evolution of modern medicine and medical facilities, the role of the environment in health care has in important respects been neglected."[1]

Some Western European countries are including green care in their mental and social health programs.[2] *Green care* is an umbrella term for health care approaches that combine traditional medical interventions with agriculture, therapeutic horticulture and gardening, landscape conservation, wilderness activities, animal-assisted therapies and/or caring for and breeding domestic animals.[3] All of these approaches draw on an understanding that nature contact is crucial for human well-being—physically, socially, spiritually and psychologically. Nature is not just a backdrop for health and healing activities, but rather a necessary part of the experience.

Within the wider research on human-nature connections, three main benefits are consistently identified. In particular, green care clients tend to exhibit:

1. improved mood, self-esteem and self-efficacy (which includes better coping) as well as reduced anger, confusion, depression and tension
2. better physical health
3. enhanced social connections and ability to bond with others.[4]

While most studies are conducted with civilian populations, anyone familiar with the struggles of former military personnel suffering from the effects of stress and post-traumatic stress (as outlined in Chapter 1) will recognize that the above-listed benefits hold important possibilities for veterans' recovery and reintegration. In these times of economic strain and austerity, as well as high rates of stress injuries and suicide amongst soldiers and veterans, it seems urgent to find adjunct methods of care to ease the transition to civilian life and to support veterans in healing from exposure to military trauma.

Overview of Green Care

In the past 100 years, many of us have come to lead increasingly urban lives that seem disconnected from nature; we often forget that we and our own bodies are nature, too. I used the words "seem disconnected," because we continue to rely on nature for all our needs: food, clothing, water, housing and electricity. Everything that surrounds us, in our homes and offices, at malls and supermarkets, comes from the Earth, even when the final forms are no longer recognizable as such. If you are reading this book in paper format, the page on which these words are printed was once a tree, and the inks are derived from vegetable sources.[5] If you are reading it as an e-book, the metals and metalloids that make up your e-reader or computer were mined from the Earth, and the plastic casing is derived from petroleum, itself the fossilized remains of plants and animals that lived millions of years ago.

The remembrance of our own nature is even found in our language, where the English word human comes originally from the Latin *humus*, which quite literally implies that humans are of the earth, soil or ground. Similarly, the Hebrew word for man, *adam*, comes from the Hebrew *ad-amah* meaning "ground." This notion of being human, as connected to the Earth and soil, points to one of the central insights of this book: that human bodies and minds are inseparable from the sensible world. With this in mind, it simply makes sense that nature provides an important context for healing.

Green Care in Europe

Approaches to green care vary within Europe, although many countries put particular emphasis on green care farms (also called *social farming* or *care farming*). The growth of care farming led the intergovernmental framework for European Cooperation in Science and Technology (COST), in 2006, to establish a working group to investigate Green Care in Agriculture (COST Action 866) as part of its Food and Agriculture program.[6] For the purpose of the group's research, Green Care in Agriculture was defined as "the [use] of agricultural farms—the animals, the plants, the garden, the forest, and the landscape—as a base for promoting human mental and physical health, as well as quality of life, for a variety of client groups."[7] Accordingly, the project's main objective was to "increase the scientific knowledge on the best practices for implementing green care in agriculture with the aim of improving human mental and physical health and the quality of life."[8]

The Netherlands, where care farming has become a comprehensive, professionalized movement, is considered to be a leader in the field. Care farming is supported by the Ministry of Agriculture, Nature and Food Quality and the Ministry of Health, and the country ensures nationwide standards through a system of training courses, education programs and certification procedures. The number of care farms in the country rose more than 1,000-fold in 10 years, from 75 in 1998 to more than 800 in 2008.[9] Today, there are more than 1,000 care farms in The Netherlands, all of which are privately owned farms that earn an income from selling agricultural products, while also offering agriculture-related health care activities. The target group of these programs has expanded in the past 15 years from its initial focus on people struggling with psychiatric difficulties and/or intellectual disabilities to include those suffering from addictions, burnout and chronic unemployment, as well as young children and older adults. The majority of participants in the Dutch programs are male,[10] which makes them interesting models to investigate since the majority of veterans in North America are also male.

In addition, or as an alternative, to medication and/or therapy, a health professional such as a doctor or psychiatrist can refer a patient to work on a care farm for a continuous period or as a weekly activity. Farmers operating a designated care farm are paid to provide this service by health care institutions, insurance plans or even directly by the customer. They also benefit from the added workers, while clients derive health benefits from working on the farm.[11]

In The Netherlands, care farming is now an important income source for many farmers, which helps offset the unpredictable nature of small-scale farming.[12] The emphasis here is that farmers, while they do take training in green care methods, are ordinary farmers, not health care professionals. And care farming clients become involved in the everyday work and life on a farm. Accordingly, the role of care farmers is providing care "on a small scale, with personal attention and individual care."[13]

There are some costs to this Dutch model of care farming, not all of which can be quantified in monetary terms. For example, the farmer needs to take extra time to plan for and guide the green care clients who come to work on the farm; it also takes time to liaise with health care providers who refer clients to the farm.[14] Some farmers need to hire additional staff to facilitate green care activities. Also, farmers often require extra insurance to host clients. There can be increased costs, too, for items such as electricity, water, food and/or gas, and the farm may need to be modified to include disabled access and customized work tools. Accordingly, it is difficult to determine what constitutes fair compensation for Dutch care farmers.[15]

Most other European countries that offer care farming and green care are doing so in a less formal way. Only Flanders (Belgium), Norway and Slovenia are moving in a similar direction to The Netherlands with the primary involvement of private farmers.[16] And even within these countries, there are important differences: while The Netherlands emphasizes economic and diversification opportunities for farmers, for example, Flanders views green care as a primarily social service.[17]

In countries such as Germany and Austria, green care remains typically the responsibility of health care professionals.[18] While ordinary farms do occasionally provide the context for green care activities, for the most part health care establishments operate their own gardens and farms. This approach to health care has a long tradition in Germany. Since the 19th century, many German social programs have incorporated participants into their daily work, with a special focus on working in the kitchen and gardens.[19] While this approach waned in the 1960s and 1970s, a new awareness of the importance of nature in human life has led to a revival of such programs. For example, the Berlin Center for Torture Victims incorporates an Intercultural Healing Garden as part of its work with victims of torture and human rights violations.[20] And today, Germany has a number of care farms, which have specific relationships with health care facilities; unlike The Netherlands, however, these farms cater to a much smaller client base and do not earn an income from their agricultural production.[21]

In the United Kingdom, there is an increasing movement for private farmers to provide green care services.[22] In the case of health care institutions offering gardening and farming activities, these services are paid out of institutional budgets, as well as through insurance, private health associations and individually by clients. Like Germany, the gardens and farms are generally small and do not profit from their agricultural production. The UK also has a growing focus on social and therapeutic horticulture.[23] This movement developed out of traditional horticulture therapy approaches but acknowledges the important role and benefit of social interactions and sense of community in the healing process.[24] There are currently more than 1,000 social and therapeutic horticulture programs in the UK providing care to more than 21,000 people per week.

In Italy, France and Ireland, green care is generally organized and provided through cooperatives, often on a volunteer basis. There is no formal institutional or government support, nor is green care regulated. In Italy, for example, many psychiatric institutions were closed in the early 1980s, which coincided with the rise of social cooperatives, many of which incorporated agricultural endeavors to assist former psychiatric patients.[25] Care farming in these countries is understood not only as a way of promoting health and well-being, but also as part of a "philosophy of social reintegration, participation and social inclusion" for supporting clients according to researchers Bettina Bock and Simon Oosting. "The goal is to re-establish the habit of working, build up knowledge and skills and build self-esteem. These aspects should eventually enable [clients] to find employment in the regular labour market and re-integrate into society."[26]

Green Care in North America

There is no organized discussion of green care in the US and Canada, particularly at national and health care levels. Indeed, some recent moves, such as the Canadian government's decision in 2009 to close prison farms, suggest a level of hostility toward green care. In Chapter 2, Keith Tidball from Cornell University confirmed that there is sometimes resistance within the military community and the US Veterans Administration to green care, something he considers to be a major challenge in his work to advocate outdoor recreation for former military personnel. For example, several years ago, Tidball worked with a group at Fort Drum to create a companion gardening program for military families, where both the deployed soldier and the family at home received an earthbox or community garden plot. This program gave the families a common experience to talk about while the soldier was away. "That worked pretty well, but there was resistance to it," Tidball explained. Indeed, he continued, a lack of support from Commanding

Officers "kills a whole line of horticultural therapy that could be very useful."[27]

I believe, however, that the veterans' stories shared in this book provide evidence of a veteran-led green care movement in North America. First Lady Michelle Obama might also be promoting a form of green care in her Let's Move campaign's emphasis on vegetable gardening. And healing gardens (also referred to as therapeutic gardens or restorative gardens) are beginning to gain popularity in some hospitals and other types of health care facilities, both for veterans and the wider community.

Since 2008, for example, the Warrior and Family Support Center (WFSC) at Fort Sam Houston in San Antonio, Texas, has operated a large therapeutic garden, complete with shrubs, trees, perennials, vegetables, a water feature and extensive walking trails. The garden is available to veterans in the WFSC treatment program and their families.[28] The plans for a new facility at the Irwin Army Community Hospital at Fort Riley, Kansas, incorporate a healing garden.[29] And to curtail stress levels amongst officers, city police in Vancouver, BC, Canada recently started a rooftop vegetable garden.[30]

The Center for Victims of Torture in Minneapolis, Minnesota, also features a garden. The Center's clients, many of whom suffer from post-traumatic stress, can wait for appointments in the garden, and many counselors also spend time there to help them cope with the stress and anguish that come from hearing stories of pain and suffering every day.[31] Many of the staff have also taken up gardening at home. Further, since trauma survivors often suffer from loneliness and isolation, the Center uses gardening "to help people connect with one another and reestablish a sense of trust."[32]

In Canada, some traumatic stress sufferers are being referred to the Homewood Health Centre in Guelph, Ontario, which prescribes horticulture therapy (both in greenhouses and outdoor gardens) as part of patients' treatment.[33]

Based on his own journey to recover from post-traumatic stress, LCol Chris Linford advocates that nature-based experiences need to be made more widely available to veterans. In 2011, he spent a week on an Outward Bound Canada Veterans' Program trip, which he described as "a significant 'pivot point' on my personal path to improved health."[34] And during a conversation with me, he further described the ways that the Outward Bound trip helped him to "return to a childlike humor and innocence."[35]

Today there is also a growing movement in the US, led by organizations such as the Farmer Veteran Coalition (FVC),[36] and by veterans themselves, to provide opportunities for former military personnel to move into farming. Farming and working outdoors offer possibilities to engage with plants and animals, nurture and cultivate new life and provide healthy food to feed other people. In addition to health gains, veterans becoming involved in farming provides succession planning for American food security, since many current farmers are expected to retire during the next 10 years. Indeed, the main emphasis of the FVC, which has helped more than 1,000 farmer veterans in the past 6 years, is that agriculture provides a viable career option for veterans. "Agriculture is not easy, and veterans have a lot of practical skills," said Tia Christopher, FVC Chief of Staff. "But they also have a huge strength due to what many of them have lived through that helps them stick it out in a very, very tough secondary career."[37]

The FVC supports farmer veterans in all areas of agriculture, ranging from small-scale organic operations to conventional ranches and farms. There are often regional differences, Tia explained, wherein veterans living in the central prairies tend to be more attracted to large-scale cattle ranching and farming, while those living on the east and west coasts are more likely to become involved in small-scale sustainable agriculture. And while the FVC emphasizes agriculture as a career option, "we really do stand behind the positive psychological effects," said Tia. "What I've found really interesting is that you hear about equine therapy, but you don't really hear about cattle therapy. And for my folks who have picked up cattle ranching, it's amazing how they've healed. People with serious injuries and so much anger about having to rebuild their lives and learn how to walk and talk again...for some of them working with the cattle has really helped them." Tia Christopher has also seen benefits for veterans with brain injuries, who can no longer do their former jobs. "They've retrained in agriculture, and not only is it now a viable career option, but it also helps them to continue to heal."

Tia also emphasized benefits for families. "Families that have been separated over years of multiple deployments become fractured and don't really know how they fit together, and they have to re-get-to-know their spouse or their dad," she explained. "And when you have folks that come together for a family farm, it actually helps heal the family. They all have a job, they all contribute, they all build the business together, face tough winters or bad harvests...I'm amazed at what I've seen that do for families."

In my own research and conversations with veterans, I have found that many are gravitating toward small-scale, often organic, farms, a trend Tia Christopher has also seen amongst farmer veterans. "Even though we have veterans representing all different schools of thought when it comes to agriculture, I've found anecdotally that the majority of veterans entering this field want to do sustainable agriculture in some way, shape or form," she told me. "They want it for their own personal health, and then that translates to what they raise for other people, what they want to sell and how they want to live."[38] And perhaps importantly, as author Sarah Elton put it, "sustainable agriculture needs people. Lots of people."[39] Indeed, a 2007 UN Food and Agriculture Organization report stated that "organic farms provide more than 30 percent more jobs per [hectare] than non-organic farms and, thus, create employment opportunities."[40] Accordingly, the work and skills training in farming activities and programs can also contribute to resolving unemployment and homelessness amongst veterans. Educational institutions are becoming involved, too; the University of Nebraska—Nebraska College of Technical Agriculture (NCTA) offers a Combat Boots to Cowboy Boots program to train veterans to become farmers, ranchers and business entrepreneurs.[41]

A number of veteran-owned farms throughout the US have become well-known in recent years for their peer-support initiatives. One example is Archi's Acres, an organic farm in Southern California run by Colin Archipley, along with his wife, Karen. Archipley is a former Marine

Corps infantry sergeant who served three tours in Iraq. Together, the Archipleys run the Veterans Sustainable Agriculture Training (VSAT) program, a six-week course in organics, hydroponics and sustainable agriculture for veterans interested in new careers as farmers.[42] In addition to teaching farming skills, such as planting and irrigation and designing a business plan to facilitate a career change for veterans, "farming offers veterans a chance to decompress," Archipley told the *New York Times*.[43] More importantly, it provides a sense of purpose. "It allows [veterans] to be physically active, be part of a unit," Colin Archipley said. "It gives them a mission statement—a responsibility to the consumer eating their food." A graduate of the Archipleys' VSAT program, Mike Hanes, who returned from Iraq suffering from post-traumatic stress, depression and a traumatic brain injury, said, "One thing I've noticed about agriculture is that you become a creator rather than a destroyer."[44]

Another prominent farmer veteran enterprise is the Veterans Farm, an organic blueberry farm in Central Florida started by Adam Burke, a US Army combat veteran and Purple Heart recipient. He returned from Iraq with a traumatic brain injury and suffering from post-traumatic stress and was urged by his psychiatrist and psychologist to find ways to alleviate his stress. Having grown up on a farm, Burke recalled that some of his best times were spent there: "I remembered being in the outdoors and enjoying working with others. I remember the sound of the birds and the mist from the sprinklers, the wind and the calming effect it had on me."[45] With help from the Farmer Veteran Coalition, Burke started the handicapped-accessible Veterans Farm, which now provides a six-month fellowship program to promote and support agro-entrepreneurship and ecological horticulture amongst veterans.

In a YouTube video, Burke told a story about sitting under a tree with a veteran who was suffering from a panic attack; the two men sat together and talked for two hours, feeling a light breeze on their skin under the shade of a tree. At the end of their conversation, the other veteran turned to Burke and said: "Adam, this is the most peace I've felt since I've been back from war. I can sit in a conference room, I can sit in a medical setting, I can see psychologists all day, but nothing compares to sitting in this chair under this tree on this farm."[46]

Still other US examples include the 15-acre Veterans' Garden in West Los Angeles, where veterans cultivate fruits and vegetables in the middle of the city and sell their produce to local restaurants.[47] And in Brockton, Massachusetts, the Veterans Administration Medical Center provides a horticulture therapy program. Twenty-four-year-old Afghanistan veteran Chris Pina said that working in the garden at the VA Center has been important for him: "I've learned a lot about plants so far, and actually I'm starting to do it at home now. I see a brighter light." Several other veterans who work in the garden described how the plant life showed them the ways that life can continue beyond their military experiences.[48]

Learning from Veterans' Stories and Experiences

Green care is producing significant results in a variety of ways for many veterans. The veterans featured in this book have described, amongst other things, the importance of meaningful service, social connections and camaraderie, regaining a sense of safety, physical activity and overall nature contact.

In examining these benefits, it is helpful to keep in mind the ways that the military, and contexts such as military academies, basic training and missions away from home, fall within the realm of what sociologist Erving Goffman named *total institutions*.[49] Such institutions provide an all-encompassing experience for those working and living inside them. In the military, service members learn very specific ways of being and acting; soldiers are taught a deep sense of discipline and to obey superiors, as well as to suppress their emotions, particularly fear and grief.[50]

Understanding the military as an institution that totally orients the lives, bodies and emotions of soldiers is helpful in making sense of the lack of purpose and feelings of loss that some describe upon leaving the military; this makes the transition to civilian life difficult. For veterans suffering from post-traumatic stress, these difficulties are compounded by the symptoms of their injury. Flashbacks and panic attacks, for example, are unpredictable, often leading to lost confidence. Experiencing a flashback and becoming incapacitated in an everyday situation, such as grocery shopping, often leads veterans to avoid such situations, to withdraw and disengage from community life. Moreover, in that the military becomes like a second family for most soldiers, leaving the military can be comparable to losing one's entire family.

With this context in mind, let's consider the main benefits veterans are finding through nature contact.

Meaningful Service

Researchers at the Medical University of Vienna have found a strong correlation between nature connectedness and meaningfulness.[51] The notion of meaningful service came up repeatedly in my conversations with veterans, who were looking for opportunities to continue serving their communities. Farming and conservation work in particular offer a variety of meaningful activities, ranging from nurturing and caring for plants and animals, to problem-solving and developing organization skills.[52] In the case of veterans who are unemployed, underemployed or living on disability benefits, such work also provides structure to their day, something to look forward to and a place to concentrate their thoughts.

Beyond the work of farms and nature conservation, however, all nature contact provides possibilities for meaningful integration into the wider community beyond the military, particularly in veterans' peer-support efforts. Recall, too, Keith Tidball's description of how hunting and fishing can sometimes bring new understanding and meaning to death. As the veterans who shared their stories with me spent time interacting with nature, all described feeling a new sense of purpose, regaining lost confidence and realizing they had a valuable role to play in their communities, which often included supporting other veterans.

Social Connections and Camaraderie

Judith Herman, clinical professor of psychiatry with expertise in trauma exposure, indicates that "disconnection from others" is a core experience associated with psychological trauma.[53] Recent research indicates that stress and isolation are harmful to human health, can lead to slower healing and magnify and multiply illness outcomes; thus, scientist and physician Esther Sternberg reflected, "positive social interactions are important buffers against stress."[54]

Peer support amongst veterans is increasingly acknowledged by veterans themselves as a fundamental aspect in easing the transition to civilian life and learning to cope with and heal from post-traumatic experiences. The veterans' experiences also reflect the ways that social support and camaraderie, particularly with other veterans, are both found and facilitated in nature settings. In many chapters in *Field Exercises*, veterans described feeling separate from the human communities in which they were living, but as they connected with others who could understand their experiences, they gained a purpose in life beyond the military and a sense of responsibility to other people, plants and animals. Nature, it seems, provides an important context for veterans to connect at the level of their shared experience.

For some, though, it is at times difficult to be part of the human community, and the wider planetary community—animals in particular—also provides support to ground their lives in the present and carry their living forward. Christian McEachern described how his dogs and horses have provided great company and important relationships, and how horses especially provide a sense of peace unrivalled by anything else in his life. Similarly, Shepherd Bliss found that his dog, Winnie, has brought great joy and playfulness back into his life. And with the Can Praxis equine therapy program, we saw how working with horses brought new insights to veterans and supported them in reconnecting with loved ones.

Regaining a Sense of Safety

Many North American veterans, and particularly those suffering from the effects of stress, describe not feeling safe once they returned home to Canada or the US. Military personnel are trained to deal with the uncertainty and unpredictability of combat by reacting with speed and aggression and by being constantly vigilant and aware of their surroundings; however, there are always elements beyond a soldier's control. Their military training, wartime and/or peacekeeping experiences are forever imprinted on their psyche and body, and become the new vantage from which they experience the world. These experiences lead many to feel constantly threatened by people and situations they encounter in daily life at home.

In my conversation with neuroscientist Kelly Lambert, she explained that, in the war zone, soldiers' brains help to protect them by making associations with certain sounds and smells. "It was absolutely adaptive and absolutely normal for them to be very vigilant about every little thing in their environment—that kept them alive," explained Lambert. "But the problem is: how do you switch from that vigilance to telling your brain, 'OK, I'm in a different environment; I'm safe; I don't need to be that hypervigilant right now'?"

Lambert believes that nature offers an environment "that optimizes the transition from a combat zone." The veterans' stories included in this book point clearly to nature as a place they feel secure, and the ways that through contact with nature they find possibilities for carrying their lives forward. Lambert told me it is important for veterans to help their brains transition to civilian life by weakening some of the associations with sounds, smells and other sensations. "And that's maybe what they're doing in some of these farming situations where it is quiet and there aren't loud noises; they're not using power tools; they're using their hands. They're having some time where they're not activating those associations," she explained.[55]

In situations where veterans work with their hands, they also activate what Lambert calls *effort-driven rewards*. In her book *Lifting Depression*, Lambert brought attention to the work of neurobiologists who speculate that, based on the large amount of brain space dedicated to hand movement, the human brain evolved as our ancestors performed tasks related to survival requiring extensive hand use, such as hunting, gathering, gardening, cooking and making clothing.[56] Lambert incorporated this research into her own argument about effort-driven rewards, in which completing tasks with our hands sends messages to the brain's pleasure center, which releases feel-good hormones. (I'm greatly simplifying Lambert's research and recommend reading her book to gain an understanding of all the various processes involved.)

So how do effort-driven rewards relate to feelings of safety? "You build associations where you're gaining control. You're exerting effort, you're making a response, and you're seeing a desired consequence," Lambert told me. "You see some immediate things: dirt is moved around, things are harvested. Some things are longer term (waiting for plants to grow), but you're using both of those hands, you're activating your brain, you're anticipating what's going to happen and then you see results."[57] These activities teach the brain that effort is related to positive consequences, and accordingly, enable veterans to gain a sense of control over the world around them. Lambert's research ties in well with Tia Christopher's comments shared in the introduction of this book, when she said, "We've found that when veterans can follow a plant cycle—when they prepare the earth, they plant the seed, they nurture it, they harvest it and they eat it or they sell it—that process in itself is healing."[58]

Physical Activity

The importance of physical activity came up often in my conversations with veterans—not the extreme pursuits that were part of military life and training—but rather moving their bodies according to their current ability, whether in gardening and farming, canoeing, horseback riding or hiking. Kelly Lambert pointed to how "most of the research suggests that if you supplement your pharmacological therapy—your drugs— with exercise or some other kind of cognitive therapy, you're going to get a better outcome." This is because effort-driven rewards and physical activities and behaviors are able to tap into more neurochemicals than any single drug, even though some of the drugs are tapping into two or three different neurochemicals, Lambert explained. "Sometimes people are so distraught, so anxious—maybe in a panic mode—that they need to be recalibrated with drugs, but it would be great if doctors and therapists were able to consider all of these as they decide what is best for the veterans."[59]

Nature Contact

The empirical studies summarized in Chapter 2 bring attention to the ways that nature contact works on a variety of interconnected levels, from influencing the production of serotonin to lowering blood pressure and increasing emotional resilience. Many veterans' descriptions of their experience reinforce this research—and in turn are supported by it.

Ecopsychologist Andy Fisher has written that our human bodies "still carry the knowledge of our buried needs, of our unactivated interactional patterns."[60] The veterans all described coming to the realization that they feel better when they are outside and interacting with nature. Each veteran's story elucidated an overwhelming sense of presence, mindfulness and awareness, as well as the calm and peace that comes with those experiences. And as described in Chapter 2, Fisher suggests that through these experiences, each veteran's body is implying its need to connect to the wider world, which is demonstrated by the shift in their experiences when they spend time in nature. Also, Kenneth Helphand, author of *Defiant Gardens*, wrote that gardens "foster a form of nonverbal communication among a person, plant and place. They offer an opportunity to nurture."[61]

Through flashbacks and panic attacks, post-traumatic stress sufferers are easily drawn into the past—a past that seems to be happening in the present. Nature contact provides an alternate sensory experience to stress reactions and/or symptoms associated with post-traumatic stress. In listening to and writing the veterans' stories, I was struck by how their experiences in the natural world have turned their attention to the ways that nature is regulated by cycles and seasons, by birth and death, by relations between animals and plants. Nature presents its own rhythm, which perhaps provides a metaphor for veterans' own struggles and journeys.

Inner Nature and Mindfulness

To this point, I have focused mainly on interactions with natural places, plants and animals—that is, nature outside the human body. But we and our bodies are nature, too. This was brought home during a conversation with Kurt Hoelting, author of *The Circumference of Home*, who is a long-time Zen practitioner and has spent a lot of time in nature as a commercial fisherman, climber and wilderness guide.[62] Kurt now runs Inside Passages, a sea kayaking guide business, which offers contemplative kayaking retreats in Alaska.[63] Most of his clients are environmental activists and religious leaders. These retreats, Kurt told me, are designed as a means for "restoring our inner habitat of heart and mind and spirit, which naturally happens when we're in nature in all kinds of ways."[64]

In collaboration with Dr. David Kearney at the Puget Sound regional VA Hospital in Seattle, Kurt also teaches Mindfulness-Based Stress Reduction (MBSR) to veterans suffering from post-traumatic stress disorder.[65] MBSR is a secular approach to mindfulness meditation based on the work of Jon Kabat-Zinn, who founded the Stress Reduction Program at the University of Massachusetts Medical School.[66] The eight-week MBSR course was initially designed for patients suffering from chronic pain who needed additional support outside the medical system. The program is now offered worldwide to many others also suffering from stress and/or pain. The course incorporates insights from meditation and gentle yoga to guide participants to work with their experience and learn relaxation skills that can be accessed even in the midst of discomfort and pain. Participants' homework is to practice mindfulness for approximately 45 minutes every day. They then come together once per week to meditate and talk about their practice, challenges and insights during the previous week. In this way, course participants reinforce and support one another's mindfulness experiences. And Kurt described that, through the MBSR course, many of the veterans in his class "come to an understanding that they have a lot more capacity than they thought they did to shift their relationship with their pain, if not eliminate the pain itself."[67]

Generally, courses are located in a room in the basement of the VA Hospital, a context he described as "pretty bleak," perhaps especially compared to the wild surroundings of his Inside Passages work. However, Kurt sees many "overlapping circles" between his kayak retreats and his MBSR work with veterans. In particular, he described both as "leading people into the vicinity of their own inner wildness and giving them some ways to navigate the complexity of that interior terrain, so that the grief can have its place at the table, the fear, the anger, all of that, as well as the wonder and all the positive things that we associate with being in a beautiful place." And, Kurt said, "Just as it's possible to be in a really gorgeous, wild place and feel really depressed, be really not present," it's possible to be in a room in the basement of the VA Hospital "and do the work of mindfulness, of sitting quietly and also drop into a place of deep presence and gratitude and buoyancy and resilience."

During our conversation, Kurt reflected on the deep interconnections between nature outside the human body and nature inside us. "Our culture tends to think of nature as being out there and something that we go out there to get. But actually, this is inside of us as much as it's outside of us," he said. "I'm blown away, actually, by how much of this same capacity for being present in a relaxed way, and at ease even in the midst of a lot of pain and distress in our lives, can happen at the VA Hospital as well as in the wilderness. So that suggests to me that it's the inner nature, inner habitat, that is the critical component here."[68]

During the MBSR course, in addition to the weekly two-hour meetings, six weeks into the course there is a full-day meditation retreat, in which participants come together to spend seven hours in silence. Most of these all-day retreats take place in the same basement room used for the veterans' weekly MBSR meetings, but Kurt once hosted such a retreat in a natural place. "And I think the benefit is pretty obvious," he said, recalling the experience: "When you get away from a place that's noisy and dark, and you get out into the fresh air, into a place where natural sound is able to make itself felt, the heart and the mind just open more easily. You can feel the boundary between self and world softening. It doesn't have that hard edge that is so often there when you're in a hospital basement somewhere. However, regardless of where you are," Kurt reflected, "you still have to do the same work of attending, of arriving, of starting where you are. And nature doesn't just do that for us. We have to do that work ourselves. It's an inside job."

In addition, over the weeks of a course, Kurt has discovered that an important human connection develops between the veterans and himself—a connection that is "a manifestation of healing nature," he said. "Our human nature wants to connect. And the primary way that we connect with nature is through each other, through our human nature: through words, through emotions, through shared experience. And when it can be linked to the wider nature around us, that amplifies our sense of being part of something much bigger than ourselves. In a strange kind of way, it's all connected. It's all very much working with healing nature."[69]

Concluding Thoughts:
Supporting Green Care in North America

In writing *Field Exercises*, I am not under the illusion that nature contact will solve or cure all veterans' problems; and I am especially interested in Kurt Hoelting's suggestion that inner nature is the critical component—perhaps this is the topic of another book. But I also agree with Keith Tidball, who told me, "Almost across the board, in every case, nature contact matters."[70] As I wrote earlier, this book is intended to gather support for North American veterans working to incorporate green care into their healing, recovery and reintegration. And I like to imagine a very near future when this wide support is possible. In each of the stories, intimate contact with nature as well as social contact with and support from other veterans helped to imbue life with new or remembered meaning. It was through intimate contact with/in nature that the veterans remembered they are part of the world, that they are anchored to the world and that they began to make sense of their experiences.

Imagine, then, if these efforts were supported at a wider societal level. If, for example, physicians, psychiatrists and counselors could prescribe veterans to work on farms or to take part in other green care activities. Over time, many veterans would likely benefit in the ways I have described. Joe Sempik, a research fellow at the University of Nottingham, has stressed that green care is differentiated from other health care approaches in its emphasis on the centrality of nature to our human being and well-being. While most health care providers underscore providing "productivity, structure and routine" for patients, clients in green care programs instead highlight that their experience of interacting with nature is most important to them, both in terms of nurturing plants and/or animals as well as developing a deeper connection with the wider world.[71]

It is time to pay attention to the stories of veterans who are finding paths through suffering and despair by connecting with nature. Their stories reveal that connecting into life—into the living—matters. It is time to fund and support veteran-led initiatives, whether in formalized ways as happens in some European countries or in more informal ways that nevertheless make these activities and experiences available to as many veterans as would like to participate. "In contrast to war," Kenneth Helphand has written, "gardens assert the dignity of life, human and nonhuman, and celebrate it."[72]

Returning to the words of Shepherd Bliss, "There's something about the healing power of the regenerative earth, the grass, the leaves, the flowers, the bees, whatever wanders in, the ants while they're doing their work, and the honeybees that don't sting." And in the words of Iraq war veteran Nathan Lewis, "There are not many fixes, and gardening's not a fix but it's an effort. It gives you a fighting chance. It keeps you in the game. It allows you to take control of your own situation, of your own destiny."

ENDNOTES

Introduction

1. Tia Christopher. Conversation with author, October 18, 2013.
2. For the purposes of this book, *nature* includes both animate and inanimate elements of nature, and *nature contact* is broadly interpreted to be any direct experiences with and interaction in the wider world, including spaces and places that might be classified as "wild" (rivers, mountains and generally rural places) as well as urban nature (parks, green spaces, backyard gardens, greenhouses, animals and even houseplants).
3. Keith Tidball. Conversation with author, September 4, 2013.
4. Some of the veterans in this book share stories about coming off medication—or even avoiding taking medication—with the support of farming and other outdoor activities. This is a personal decision that individuals should discuss with health professionals. For many others, medication continues to be an essential part of their everyday life and healing.
5. Edward Tick. *War and the Soul: Healing Our Nation's Veterans from Post-traumatic Stress Disorder*. Quest, 2005, p. 5.
6. Peter Raymont, director. *Shake Hands with the Devil: The Journey of Roméo Dallaire*. Video, Canadian Broadcasting Corporation, White Pine Pictures, Société Radio Canada, 2004.
7. Viktor E. Frankl. *Man's Search for Meaning*, with a new foreword by Harold S. Kushner. Beacon, 1959/2006.
8. Ibid., pp. 39–40.
9. Donald Creighton. *Harold Adams Innis: Portrait of a Scholar*. University of Toronto, 1957, p. 63.
10. Kenneth Helphand. *Defiant Gardens: Making Gardens in Wartime*. Trinity University, 2006.
11. Ibid., p. 48.
12. Shell-shock was the term used during World War I for what is now referred to as post-traumatic stress disorder. See Chapter 1 for a discussion of the changing terminology and understanding of combat-related stress and distress.

13. Eva M. Selhub and Alan C. Logan. *Your Brain on Nature: The Science of Nature's Influence on Your Health, Happiness, and Vitality.* Wiley, 2012, p. 153.

14. Charles A. Lewis. *Green Nature/Human Nature: The Meaning of Plants in Our Lives.* University of Illinois, 1996; Paula Diane Relf. "Agriculture and Health Care: The Care of Plants and Animals for Therapy and Rehabilitation in the United States" in Jan Hassink and Majken van Dijk, eds. *Farming for Health: Green-Care Farming across Europe and the United States of America.* Springer, 2006; Richard Louv. *Last Child in the Woods: Saving Our Children from Nature-deficit Disorder,* updated and expanded ed. Algonquin, 2008.

15. Elizabeth R. Messer Diehl. "Gardens that Heal" in L. Buzzell and C. Chalquist, eds. *Ecotherapy: Healing with Nature in Mind.* Sierra Club, 2009; Ingrid Söderback, Marianne Söderström and Elisabeth Schälander. "Horticultural Therapy: The 'Healing Garden' and Gardening in Rehabilitation Measures at Danderyd Hospital Rehabilitation Clinic, Sweden." *Developmental Neurorehabilitation* Vol. 7 (2004), pp. 245–60.

16. Relf, "Agriculture and Health Care," p. 315.

17. Government of Canada. *Veterans' Land Act* R.S.C. 1970, c. V-4." [online]. [cited August 27, 2013]. laws-lois.justice.gc.ca/PDF/V-1.5.pdf; *The Canadian Encyclopedia.* "Veterans' Land Act." [online]. [cited August 27, 2013]. thecanadianencyclopedia.com/articles/veterans-land-act.

18. Tadzio Richards. "Landmine in a Rucksack: Homecoming Soldiers Aren't Necessarily Home Free." *Alberta Views,* June 2010, p. 42.

Chapter 1

1. Used with permission of both author and editor. Maxine Hong Kingston, ed. *Veterans of War, Veterans of Peace.* Koa, 2006, pp. 413–14, vowvop.org.

2. For many civilians, the word *veteran* invokes the image of men from a different generation: an elderly man, perhaps a father or grandfather, who served in World War II. But the picture of veterans in North America has changed. While most continue to be male (in the US, 93% are male; in Canada, 88% are male), many post-9/11 veterans are at the beginning of their adult life, from their late teens to early 20s, and many others are in their 30s and 40s. Some similarities might be drawn to the Vietnam War, in which young males in late adolescence or early adulthood who were still forming their identities made up most of the US infantry.

3. US Department of Labor, Bureau of Labor Statistics. "Employment Situation of Veterans News Release," March 20, 2013. [online]. [cited August 20, 2013]. bls.gov/news.release/archives/vet_03202013.htm.

4. Veterans Affairs Canada Research Directorate. *Income Study: Regular Force Veteran Report,* January 4, 2011. [online]. [cited September 13, 2013].

publications.gc.ca/collections/collection_2011/acc-vac/V32-230-2011-eng
.pdf.

5. Veterans Affairs Canada. "Providing Timely and Effective Support to
   Homeless Veterans." [online]. [cited September 13, 2013]. veterans.gc.ca
   /eng/department/reports/ovo-response/ovo-homeless.

6. Judy Jackson. *War in the Mind*. Film, TVO and Judy Films BC Inc., 2011.
   [online]. [cited November 12, 2011]. docstudio.tvo.org/story/war-mind.

7. Shannon Jones. "Homelessness Soars among US Iraq and Afghanistan War
   Veterans." *World Socialist Web Site*, December 31, 2012. [online]. [cited September 13, 2013]. wsws.org/en/articles/2012/12/31/vets-d31.html.

8. LCol Chris Linford. *Warrior Rising*. Friesen, 2013, p. 309.

9. The term *moral injury* is becoming a common alternative to post-traumatic
   stress disorder. A detailed discussion of terminology follows later in this
   chapter.

10. Shepherd Bliss. Conversation with author, July 11, 2013.

11. Raymond Monsour Scurfield and Katherine Theresa Platoni. "Myths and
    Realities about War, Its Impact, and Healing" in Raymond Monsour Scur-
    field and Katherine Theresa Platoni, eds. *War Trauma and Its Wake: Ex-
    panding the Circle of Healing*. Routledge, 2012.

12. The Standing Senate Committee on National Security and Defence. *Oc-
    cupational Stress Injuries: The Need for Understanding*, Ottawa, June, 2003.
    [online]. [cited November 2, 2011]. parl.gc.ca/Content/SEN/Committee
    /372/vete/rep/rep14jun03-e.pdf.

13. Jackson, *War in the Mind*.

14. Linford, *Warrior Rising*, p. 306.

15. Jackson, *War in the Mind*.

16. Jonathan Shay. "Learning about Combat Stress from Homer's *Iliad*."
    Journal of Traumatic Stress, Vol. 4#4 (October 1991), p. 562.

17. Herodotus, trans. George Rawlinson. *The History of Herodotus*. Vol III.
    D. Appleton & Company, 1866, p. 414.

18. Tick, *War and the Soul*, p. 99.

19. Terri Tanielian and Lisa H. Jaycox, eds. *Invisible Wounds of War: Psychologi-
    cal and Cognitive Injuries, Their Consequences, and Services to Assist Recovery*.
    Rand, 2008.

20. Caroline Alexander. "The Shock of War: World War I troops were the first
    to be diagnosed with shell shock, an injury—by any name—still wreaking
    havoc." *Smithsonian Magazine* #41 (September 2010). [online]. [cited Sep-
    tember 13, 2011]. smithsonianmag.com/history-archaeology/The-Shock
    -of-War.html?c=y&story=fullstory.

21. Friedhelm Lamprecht and Martin Sack. "Posttraumatic Stress Disorder
    Revisited." *Psychosometric Medicine* Vol. 64#2 (March/April 2002), p. 224.

22. Judith L. Herman. *Trauma and Recovery: The Aftermath of Violence—From Domestic Abuse to Political Terror.* Basic, 1997; Mel Singer. "Transforming the Trauma of War in Combat Veterans" in Marianne Bussey and Judith Bula Wise, eds. *Trauma Transformed: An Empowerment Response.* Columbia, 2007.

23. *Jon Nordheimer.* "Postwar Shock Besets Ex-G.I.'s: Postwar Shock Is Found to Beset Veterans Returning from the War in Vietnam." *New York Times,* August 21, 1972, p. 1 (2 pages).

24. R. F. Mollica at al. "Mental Health in Complex Emergencies." *The Lancet,* Vol. 364#9450 (December 4, 2004), pp. 2058–67.

25. Robert M. Poole. "The Pathway Home Makes Inroads in Treating PTSD: An innovative California facility offers hope to combatants with post-traumatic stress disorder and brain injuries." *Smithsonian Magazine* #41 (September 2010). [online]. [cited September 13, 2011]. smithsonianmag .com/people-places/Learning-How-to-Treat-PTSD.html.

26. Art Harris. "Team Combs City Streets to Salvage 'Nam Veterans." *Washington Post,* February 24, 1980, p. A1 (3 pages).

27. Herbert Hendin and Ann Pollinger Haas. "Vietnam Veterans' Trauma." *New York Times,* November 11, 1984, p. 234.

28. Sally Satel. "PTSD's Diagnostic Trap." *Policy Review* #165 (February 1, 2011), pp. 41–53.

29. Richard J. McNally. "Progress and Controversy in the Study of Post-traumatic Stress Disorder." *Annual Review of Psychology* Vol. 54 (2003), pp. 229–52.

30. "Fire chiefs, union, seek federal PTSD help," *CBC News Online,* October 4, 2011. [online]. [cited October 4, 2011]. cbc.ca/news/canada/calgary/story /2011/10/04/calgary-fire-stress-disorder.html; Colin Freeze. "Hike in stress-disorder claims by Mounties raises questions for policy makers." *Globe and Mail,* August 18, 2011. [online]. [cited September 20, 2011]. theglobeandmail.com/news/national/hike-in-stress-disorder-claims-by -mounties-raises-questions-for-policy-makers/article2123341.

31. Herman, *Trauma and Recovery.*

32. Alastair Ager, "Psychosocial Needs in Complex Emergencies." *The Lancet* Vol. 360 (2002), p. s43.

33. Lamprecht and Sack, "Posttraumatic Stress Disorder Revisited."

34. Ibid.; Satel, "PTSD's Diagnostic Trap."

35. David M. Benedek. "Posttraumatic Stress Disorder from Vietnam to Today: The Evolution of Understanding during Eugene Brody's Tenure at the Journal of Nervous and Mental Disease." *The Journal of Nervous and Mental Disease* Vol. 199 (2011), pp. 544–52.

36. Ariel Eytan et al. "Determinants of Postconflict Symptoms in Albanian Kosovars." *Journal of Nervous and Mental Disease* Vol. 192 (2004), pp. 664–71.

37. Operational Stress Injury Social Support. "PEER SUPPORT— Leave None Behind," 2012. [online]. [cited October 25, 2013]. osiss.ca/en/index .html.

38. The Standing Senate Committee on National Security and Defence, *Occupational Stress Injuries*, p. 7.

39. James Hillman. *A Terrible Love of War*. Penguin, 2004, p. 62.

40. Shepherd Bliss. *Shepherd Bliss Speaks at Farmer-Veteran Benefit*. Film, September 20, 2008. [online]. [cited July 20, 2011]. youtube.com/watch?v=-7fj qw2T63E.

41. Shepherd Bliss. Conversation with author, July 28, 2011.

42. Joe Klein. "Can Service Save Us?" *TIME Magazine*, June 20, 2013. [online]. [cited June 24, 2013]. nation.time.com/2013/06/20/can-service-save-us/.

43. Religion & Ethics Newsweekly. *Jonathan Shay Extended Interview*, PBS, May 28, 2010. [online]. [cited July 25, 2013]. pbs.org/wnet/religionand ethics/?p=6384.

44. Andy Fisher. "To Praise Again: Phenomenology and the Project of Ecopsychology." *Spring Journal* #75 (2006), pp. 153–74.

45. Benedek. "Posttraumatic Stress Disorder from Vietnam to Today"; M. Hewson. "Horticultural Therapy and Post Traumatic Stress Recovery." *Journal of Therapeutic Horticulture*, Vol. XII (2001), pp. 44–47; Lamprecht and Sack, "Posttraumatic Stress Disorder Revisited."

46. Jackson, *War in the Mind*.

47. Richard J. Ross et al. "Sleep Disturbance as the Hallmark of Posttraumatic Stress Disorder." *American Journal of Psychiatry* Vol. 146 (1989), p. 700.

48. J. Rosen et al. "Concurrent Posttraumatic Stress Disorder in Psychogeriatric Patients." *Journal of Geriatric Psychiatry and Neurology* Vol. 2 (1989), pp. 65–69.

49. Jackson, *War in the Mind*.

50. Rick MacInnes-Rae. "A Brigadier-General's Dispatch (a conversation with Brigadier General Richard Giguere)," *Dispatches* [radio program], October 26, 2011. [online]. [cited October 28, 2011]. cbc.ca/dispatches/episode /2011/10/26/october-27-31-from-kabul---freetown-sierra-leone---zimbab we---chiquitania-bolivia/.

51. Linford, *Warrior Rising*, p. xvi.

52. Ibid., pp. 307–8.

53. Monica Culic. Conversation with author, January 12, 2010.

54. Penny Coleman. *Flashback: Posttraumatic Stress Disorder, Suicide, and the Lessons of War*. Beacon, 2006, p. 5.

55. Vietnam Veterans Association of Australia. "Massive Suicide Rate for Vietnam Veterans' Children," Media Release, August 7, 2000. [online]. [cited September 13, 2011]. vvaa.org.au/media12.htm. See also, for example: Catherine Panter-Brick et al. "Violence, Suffering, and Mental Health in Afghanistan: A School-based Survey." *The Lancet* Vol. 374 (2009),

pp. 807–816; Theresa Stichick Betancourt and Kashif Tanveer Khan. "The Mental Health of Children Affected by Armed Conflict: Protective Processes and Pathways to Resilience." *International Review of Psychiatry* Vol. 20 (2008), pp. 317–28.

56. Daniel S. Weiss et al. "The Prevalence of Lifetime and Partial Posttraumatic Stress Disorder in Vietnam Theater Veterans." *Journal of Traumatic Stress* Vol. 5 (1992), pp. 365–76.

57. Patricia B. Sutker et al. "Cognitive Deficits and Psychopathology among Former Prisoners of War and Combat Veterans of the Korean Conflict." *American Journal of Psychiatry* Vol. 148 (1991), pp. 67–72.

58. Mortality rate refers to the ratio of deaths within a specific population.

59. Eric F. Crawford et al. "Predicting Mortality in Veterans with Posttraumatic Stress Disorder Thirty Years after Vietnam." *The Journal of Nervous and Mental Disease* Vol. 197 (2009), pp. 260–65.

60. Jun Shigemura and Soichiro Nomura. "Mental Health Issues of Peacekeeping Workers." *Psychiatry and Clinical Neurosciences* Vol. 56 (2002), pp. 483–91.

61. Wanderson F. Souza et al. "Posttraumatic Stress Disorder in Peacekeepers: A Meta-Analysis." *Journal of Nervous and Mental Disease* Vol. 199 (2011), pp. 309–12.

62. Ibid., p. 309.

63. Shigemura and Nomura, "Mental Health Issues of Peacekeeping Workers," p. 486.

64. Tanielian and Jaycox, *Invisible Wounds of War.*

65. Jackson, *War in the Mind.*

66. Raymont, *Shake Hands with the Devil.*

67. Jackson, *War in the Mind.*

68. James Dao and Andrew W. Lehren. "Baffling Rise in Suicides Plagues the U.S. Military." *New York Times,* May 15, 2013. [online]. [cited May 20, 2013]. nytimes.com/2013/05/16/us/baffling-rise-in-suicides-plagues-us-military .html.

69. Craig J. Bryan and Tracy A. Clemans. "Repetitive Traumatic Brain Injury, Psychological Symptoms, and Suicide Risk in a Clinical Sample of Deployed Military Personnel." *JAMA Psychiatry* Vol. 70 (2013), pp. 686–91.

70. Ibid.

71. Cynthia A. LeardMann et al. "Risk Factors Associated with Suicide in Current and Former US Military Personnel." *Journal of the American Medical Association* Vol. 310 (2013), pp. 496–506.

72. James Dao. "Deployment Factors Are Not Related to Rise in Military Suicides, Study Finds." *New York Times,* August 6, 2013. [online]. [cited August 8, 2013]. nytimes.com/2013/08/07/us/deployment-factors-found -not-related-to-military-suicide-spike.html.

73. Janet Kemp and Robert Bossarte. *Suicide Data Report, 2012*. US Department of Veterans Affairs. [online]. [cited June 25, 2013]. va.gov/opa/docs /Suicide-Data-Report-2012-final.pdf.

74. Klein, "Can Service Save Us?"

75. Kathleen Harris. "Mental Health Issues for Soldiers, Police Up 47% since 2008." *CBC News Online*, May 1, 2013. [online]. [cited June 25, 2013]. cbc.ca /news/politics/story/2013/05/01/pol-ptsd-cases-double.html.

76. David Boulos and Mark Zamorski. "Deployment-related Mental Disorders among Canadian Forces Personnel Deployed in Support of the Mission in Afghanistan, 2001–2008." *Canadian Medical Association Journal* Vol. 185 (2013), pp. E545–52.

77. Ibid., p. E551.

78. Chris Cobb. "Military Study into Mental Injury Underplays Problem, Say Experts. *Ottawa Citizen*, July 2, 2013. [online]. [cited July 4, 2013]. ottawacitizen.com/news/Military+study+into+mental+injury+under plays+problem+experts/8606089/story.html.

79. Julian Sher. "One-quarter of Canadian soldiers return from Afghanistan with mental-health problems." *Globe and Mail*, May 30, 2011. [online]. [cited June 15, 2011]. theglobeandmail.com/news/national/one-quarter -of-canadian-soldiers-return-from-afghanistan-with-mental-health -problems/article2040698/.

80. "Domestic violence up in Canadian military families: Rates spike after Afghanistan missions." *CBC News Online*, March 31, 2011. [online]. [cited September 4, 2011]. cbc.ca/news/canada/new-brunswick/story/2011/03/30 /canadian-forces-military-domestic-violence-post-traumatic-stress-dis order.html.

81. In August 2012, the Canadian Armed Forces conducted its first survey into military sexual violence since 1998, with the results expected to be published in fall 2013.

82. Department of Defense Sexual Assault and Prevention Response. *Department of Defense Annual Report on Sexual Assault in the Military*, Fiscal Year 2012, Volume 1. [online]. [cited June 15, 2013]. sapr.mil/public/docs /reports/FY12_DoD_SAPRO_Annual_Report_on_Sexual_Assault -VOLUME_ONE.pdf, p. 2.

83. Ibid., p. 12.

84. Michael Wong. "Afterword: The Veteran Writers Group" in Kingston, ed. *Veterans of War, Veterans of Peace*, p. 210, vowvop.org.

85. Klein, "Can Service Save Us?"

86. Jackson, *War in the Mind*.

87. Scott Maxwell. Conversation with author, June 27, 2013.

88. Jo Barton and Jules Pretty. "What Is the Best Dose of Nature and Green Exercise for Improving Mental Health? A Multi-Study Analysis."

Environmental Science & Technology Vol. 44 (2010), pp. 3947–55; Valerie F. Gladwell et al. "The Great Outdoors: How a Green Exercise Environment Can Benefit All." *Extreme Physiology & Medicine* Vol. 2 (2013); Emna Diamant and Andrew Waterhouse. "Gardening and Belonging: Reflections on How Social and Therapeutic Horticulture May Facilitate Health, Well-being and Inclusion." *British Journal of Occupational Therapy* Vol. 73 (2010), pp. 84–88.

89. Kelly Lambert. *Lifting Depression: A Neuroscientist's Hands-on Approach to Activating your Brain's Healing Power.* Basic, 2008, p. 74.

90. Shay, "Learning about Combat Stress," p. 578.

91. Religion & Ethics Newsweekly, *Jonathan Shay Extended Interview.*

Chapter 2

1. Theodore Roszak. *The Voice of the Earth: An Exploration of Ecopsychology,* 2nd Edition. Phanes, 2001, p. 14.

2. Louv, *Last Child in the Woods*; Esther M. Sternberg. *Healing Spaces: The Science of Place and Well-Being.* Harvard, 2009.

3. Robert Greenway. "The Wilderness Experience as Therapy: We've Been Here Before" in Linda Buzzell and Craig Chalquist, eds. *Ecotherapy: Healing with Nature in Mind.* Sierra Club , 2009.

4. Diehl, "Gardens that Heal."

5. Jules Pretty. "How Nature Contributes to Mental and Physical Health." *Spirituality and Health International* Vol. 5#2 (June 2004), pp. 68–78.

6. Francesco Di Iacovo and Deirdre O'Connor, eds. *Supporting Policies for Social Farming in Europe: Progressing Multifunctionality in Responsive Rural Areas.* Press Service srl, 2009. [online]. [cited August 16, 2011]. sofar.unipi.it/index_file/arsia_So.Far-EU_def.pdf.

7. Louv, *Last Child in the Woods.*

8. Harold F. Searles. *The Nonhuman Environment: In Normal Development and in Schizophrenia.* International Universities, 1960, p. 3.

9. Ibid., p. 53.

10. Harold F. Searles. "Unconscious Processes in Relation to the Environmental Crisis." *Psychoanalytic Review* Vol. 59 (1972), p. 368.

11. For example, Sjerp de Vries et al. "Natural Environments–Healthy Environments? An Exploratory Analysis of the Relationship between Greenspace and Health." *Environment and Planning A* Vol. 35 (2003), pp. 1717–31; Patrik Grahn and Ulrika A. Stigsdotter. "Landscape Planning and Stress." *Urban Forestry & Urban Greening* Vol. 2 (2003), pp. 1–18; Jolanda Maas et al. "Green Space, Urbanity, and Health: How Strong Is the Relation?" *Journal of Epidemiology and Community Health* Vol. 60 (2006), pp. 587–92; Mind. *Ecotherapy: The Green Agenda for Mental Health*, May, 2007. [on-

line]. [cited October 28, 2013]. mind.org.uk/media/211255/Ecotherapy
_The_green_agenda_for_mental_health.pdf; Richard Mitchell and
Frank Popham. "Greenspace, Urbanity and Health: Relationships in En-
gland." *Journal of Epidemiology and Community Health* Vol. 61 (2007),
pp. 681–83; Jules Pretty, Jo Peacock and Rachel Hine. "Green Exercise:
The Benefits of Activities in Green Places." *The Biologist* Vol. 53 (2006),
pp. 143–48; Jules Pretty et al. "Green Exercise in the UK Countryside: Effects on Health and Psychological Well-Being, and Implications for Policy
and Planning." *Journal of Environmental Planning and Management* Vol. 50
(2007), pp. 211–31; Richard M. Ryan et al."Vitalizing Effects of Being Outdoors and in Nature." *Journal of Environmental Psychology* Vol. 30 (2010),
pp. 159–68; T. Sugiyama et al. "Associations of Neighbourhood Greenness
with Physical and Mental Health: Do Walking, Social Coherence and Local Social Interaction Explain the Relationships?" *Journal of Epidemiology
and Community Health* Vol. 62 (2008); Roger S. Ulrich et al. "Stress Recovery during Exposure to Natural and Urban Environments." *Journal of
Environmental Psychology* Vol. 11 (1991), pp. 231–48; Anne E. van den Berg,
Terry Hartig and Henk Staats. "Preference for Nature in Urbanized Societies: Stress, Restoration, and the Pursuit of Sustainability." *Journal of Social
Issues* Vol. 63 (2007), pp. 79–96.

12. Roger S. Ulrich. "View through a Window May Influence Recovery from
    Surgery." *Science* Vol. 224 (1984), pp. 420–21.

13. E. O. Moore. "A Prison Environment's Effect on Health Care Service De-
    mands." *Journal of Environmental Systems* Vol. 11 (1981), pp. 17–34.

14. Rachel Kaplan. "The Nature of the View from Home: Psychological Bene
    fits." *Environment and Behavior* Vol. 33 (2001), pp. 507–42.

15. de Vries et al., "Natural Environments—Healthy Environments?"

16. Rachel Sebba. "The Landscapes of Childhood: The Reflection of Child-
    hood's Environment in Adult Memories and in Children's Attitudes." *Envi-
    ronment and Behavior* Vol. 23 (1991), pp. 395–422.

17. Inger Jonasson, Bertil Marklund and Cathrine Hildingh. "Working in a
    Training Garden: Experiences of Patients with Neurological Damage."
    Australian Occupational Therapy Journal Vol. 54 (2007), pp. 266–72; Lucie
    Shanahan, Lindy McAllister and Michael Curtain. "Wilderness Adven-
    ture Therapy and Cognitive Rehabilitation: Joining Forces for Youth with
    TBI." *Brain Injury* Vol. 23 (2009), pp. 1054–64; Alexandra J. Walker et al.
    "Cognitive Rehabilitation after Severe Traumatic Brain Injury: A Pilot Pro-
    gramme of Goal Planning and Outdoor Adventure Course Participation."
    Brain Injury Vol. 19 (2005), pp. 1237–41; Ingeborg Eikenæs, Tore Gude and
    Asle Hoffart. "Integrated Wilderness Therapy for Avoidant Personality
    Disorder." *Nordic Journal of Psychiatry* Vol. 60 (2006), pp. 275–81; Andrea

Faber Taylor, Frances E. Kuo and William C. Sullivan. "Coping with ADD: The Surprising Connection to Green Play Settings." *Environment and Behavior* Vol. 33 (2001), pp. 54–77.

18. Terry Hartig et al., "Tracking Restoration in Natural and Urban Field Settings." *Journal of Environmental Psychology* Vol. 23 (2003), pp. 109–23.

19. Mind, *Ecotherapy*.

20. Hartig et al., "Tracking Restoration in Natural and Urban Field Settings," p. 122.

21. Jenny Roe and Peter Aspinall. "The Restorative Benefits of Walking in Urban and Rural Settings in Adults with Good and Poor Mental Health." *Health & Place* Vol. 17 (2011), pp. 103–13.

22. Terry Hartig and Henk Staats. "The Need for Psychological Restoration as a Determinant of Environmental Preferences." *Journal of Environmental Psychology* Vol. 26 (2006), pp. 215–26.

23. Terry Hartig, Ralph Catalano and Michael Ong. "Cold Summer Weather, Constrained Restoration, and the Use of Antidepressants in Sweden." *Journal of Environmental Psychology* Vol. 27 (2007), pp. 107–16.

24. Ina H. Hahn et al. "Does Outdoor Work during the Winter Season Protect Against Depression and Mood Difficulties?" *Scandinavian Journal of Work, Environment & Health* Vol. 37 (2011), pp. 446–49.

25. Ulrika K. Stigsdotter et al. "Health Promoting Outdoor Environments—Associations between Green Space, and Health, Health-related Quality of Life and Stress Based on a Danish National Representative Survey." *Scandinavian Journal of Public Health* Vol. 38 (2010), pp. 411–17.

26. Ke-Tsung Han. "Influence of Limitedly Visible Leafy Indoor Plants on the Psychology, Behavior, and Health of Students at a Junior High School in Taiwan." *Environment and Behavior* Vol. 41 (2009), pp. 658–92.

27. K. Dijkstra, M. E. Pieterse and A. Pruyn. "Stress-reducing Effects of Indoor Plants in the Built Healthcare Environment: The Mediating Role of Perceived Attractiveness." *Preventive Medicine* Vol. 47 (2008), pp. 279–83.

28. David N. Cole and Troy E. Hall. "Experiencing the Restorative Components of Wilderness Environments: Does Congestion Interfere and Does Length of Exposure Matter?" *Environment and Behavior* Vol. 42 (2010), pp. 806–23.

29. Stephen Kaplan. "The Restorative Benefits of Nature: Toward an Integrative Framework." *Journal of Environmental Psychology* Vol. 15 (1995), pp. 169–82.

30. R. Kaplan, "The Nature of the View from Home"; S. Kaplan, "The Restorative Benefits of Nature."

31. Ulrich et al., "Stress Recovery during Exposure to Natural and Urban Environments."

32. van den Berg, Hartig and Staats, "Preference for Nature in Urbanized Societies."

33. Jennifer Davis-Berman and Dene S. Berman. "The Wilderness Therapy Program: An Empirical Study of Its Effects with Adolescents in an Outpatient Setting." *Journal of Contemporary Psychotherapy* Vol. 19 (1989), pp. 271–81.

34. Christine Lynn Norton. "Into the Wilderness—A Case Study: The Psychodynamics of Adolescent Depression and the Need for a Holistic Intervention." *Clinical Social Work Journal* Vol. 38 (2010), pp. 226–35.

35. Stephen Becker. "Wilderness Therapy: Ethical Considerations for Mental Health Professionals." *Child & Youth Care Forum* Vol. 39 (2010), pp. 47–61.

36. Keith C. Russell. "Brat Camp, Boot Camp, or ....? Exploring Wilderness Therapy Program Theory." *Journal of Adventure Education & Outdoor Learning* Vol. 6 (2006), pp. 51–67.

37. Christian Itin. "Adventure Therapy and the Addictive Process." *Journal of Leisurability* Vol. 22 (1995), pp. 29–37.

38. Keith C. Russell and Jen Farnum. "A Concurrent Model of the Wilderness Therapy Process." *Journal of Adventure Education & Outdoor Learning* Vol. 4 (2007), pp. 39–55; Russell, "Brat camp, boot camp, or ....?"

39. Greenway, "The Wilderness Experience as Therapy."

40. Louv, *Last Child in the Woods*, p. 32.

41. Andrea Faber Taylor and Frances E. Kuo. "Is Contact with Nature Important for Healthy Child Development? State of the Evidence" in C. Spencer and M. Blades, eds. *Children and Their Environments: Learning, Using and Designing Spaces.* Cambridge, 2006.

42. Faber Taylor, Kuo and Sullivan, "Coping with ADD."

43. Janet E. Dyment. *Gaining Ground: The Power and Potential of School Ground Greening in the Toronto District School Board.* Evergreen, 2005. [online]. [cited March 26, 2012]. evergreen.ca/docs/res/Gaining-Ground.pdf; Anne C. Bell and Janet E. Dyment. *Grounds for Action: Promoting Physical Activity through School Ground Greening in Canada.* Evergreen, 2006. [online]. [cited March 26, 2012]. evergreen.ca/docs/res/Grounds-For-Action.pdf.

44. Nancy M. Wells. "At Home with Nature: Effects of 'Greenness' on Children's Cognitive Functioning." *Environment and Behavior* Vol. 32 (2000), p. 793.

45. Ibid., p. 781.

46. Ibid., p. 790.

47. Patrick Mooney and P. Lenore Nicell. "The Importance of Exterior Environment for Alzheimer's Residents: Effective Care and Risk Management." *Healthcare Management Forum* Vol. 5 (1992), pp. 23–29.

48. Susan Rodiek. "Influence of an Outdoor Garden on Mood and Stress in Older Persons." *Journal of Therapeutic Horticulture* Vol. 13 (2002), pp. 13–21.

49. Carol Wilkie. "Studying the Outdoors to Stimulate Mental Health." *Nursing & Residential Care* Vol. 15 (2013), pp. 223–24.

50. Annakarin Olsson et al. "Persons with Early-stage Dementia Reflect on Being Outdoors: A Repeated Interview Study." *Aging & Mental Health* Vol. 17 (2013), pp. 793–800, doi: 10.1080/13607863.2013.801065.

51. C. Colston Burrell. "Plants with Power: The Good Scents and Benefits of Using Plants." *Landscape Architecture Magazine* Vol. 90 (2000), pp. 18–19.

52. Mingwang Liu, Eunhee Kim and Richard Mattson. "Physiological and Emotional Influences of Cut Flower Arrangements and Lavender Fragrance on University Students." *Journal of Therapeutic Horticulture* Vol. 14 (2003), pp. 18–27.

53. Diehl, "Gardens that Heal."

54. Diana Beresford-Kroeger. *Arboretum America: A Philosophy of the Forest.* University of Michigan, 2003.

55. Erich Fromm. *The Heart of Man: Its Genius for Good and Evil*. Harper & Row, 1964.

56. Edward O. Wilson. *Biophilia: The Human Bond with Other Species.* Harvard, 1984; Edward O. Wilson. "Biophilia and the Conservation Ethic" in Stephen R. Kellert and Edward O. Wilson, eds. *The Biophilia Hypothesis.* Island, 1993.

57. Daniel Goleman. *Ecological Intelligence: The Hidden Impacts of What We Buy.* Broadway, 2010, p. 43; Howard Gardner. *Frames of Mind: The Theory of Multiple Intelligences.* Basic, 1983.

58. Fisher, "To Praise Again," pp. 153–54.

59. Andy Fisher. *Radical Ecopsychology: Psychology in the Service of Life*, 2nd ed. State University of New York, 2013, p. 205.

60. Ibid., p. xiii.

61. Fisher, "To Praise Again," p. 155–56.

62. Andy Fisher. Conversation with author, October 7, 2011.

63. Lambert, *Lifting Depression*, p. 243.

64. Kelly Lambert. Conversation with author, December 13, 2012.

65. Graham Rook and Laura Brunet. "Give Us This Day Our Daily Germs." *The Biologist* Vol. 49 (2002), pp. 145–49.

66. M. E. O'Brien et al. "SRL172 (Killed Mycobacterium Vaccae) in Addition to Standard Chemotherapy Improves Quality of Life without Affecting Survival, in Patients with Advanced Non-small-cell Lung Cancer: Phase III Results." *Annals of Oncology* Vol. 15 (2004), pp. 906–14.

67. C. A. Lowry et al. "Identification of an Immune-Responsive Mesolimbocortical Serotonergic System: Potential Role in Regulation of Emotional Behavior." *Neuroscience* Vol. 146 (2007), pp. 756–72.

68. G. Aghajanian and R-J. Liu. "Serotonin (5-Hydroxytryptamine; 5-HT): CNS Pathways and Neurophysiology." *Encyclopedia of Neuroscience* (2009), pp. 715–22.

69. Medical News Today. "Soil Bacteria Work in Similar Way to Antidepressants," April 2, 2007. [online]. [cited August 27, 2013]. medicalnewstoday .com/articles/66840.php.

70. Dorothy M. Matthews and Susan M. Jenks. "Ingestion of *Mycobacterium Vaccae* Decreases Anxiety-related Behavior and Improves Learning in Mice." *Behavioural Processes* Vol. 96 (2013), pp. 27–35.

71. Kaplan, "The Restorative Benefits of Nature."

72. Hartig et al., "Tracking Restoration in Natural and Urban Field Settings."

73. Frances E. Kuo and William C. Sullivan. "Aggression and Violence in the Inner City: Effects of Environment via Mental Fatigue." *Environment and Behavior* Vol. 33 (2001), pp. 543–71.

74. Erika Friedmann and Heesook Son. "The Human-Companion Animal Bond: How Humans Benefit." *Veterinary Clinics of North America: Small Animal Practice* Vol. 39 (2009), pp. 293–326.

75. Erika Friedmann and Sue A. Thomas. "Pet Ownership, Social Support, and One-year Survival after Acute Myocardial Infarction in the Cardiac Arrhythmia Suppression Trial (CAST)." *American Journal of Cardiology* Vol. 76 (1995), pp. 1213–17.

76. Andreas O. M. Hoffmann et al. "Dog-assisted Intervention Significantly Reduces Anxiety in Hospitalized Patients with Major Depression." *European Journal of Integrative Medicine* Vol. 1 (2009), pp. 145–48.

77. Norine Bardill and Sally Hutchinson. "Animal-assisted Therapy With Hospitalized Adolescents." *Journal of Child and Adolescent Psychiatric Nursing* Vol. 10 (1997), pp. 17–24; Janet Eggiman. "Cognitive-behavioral Therapy: A Case Report—Animal-assisted Therapy." *Topics in Advanced Practice Nursing eJournal* Vol. 6 (2006); Liat Hamama et al. "Preliminary Study of Group Intervention along with Basic Canine Training among Traumatized Teenagers: A 3-month Longitudinal Study." *Children and Youth Services Review* Vol. 33 (2011), pp. 1975–80.

78. Hamama et al., "Preliminary Study of Group Intervention."

79. Carie Braun et al. "Animal-assisted Therapy as a Pain Relief Intervention for Children." *Complementary Therapies in Clinical Practice* Vol. 15 (2009), pp. 105–9.

80. Hilde Hauge et al. "Equine-assisted Activities and the Impact on Perceived Social Support, Self-esteem and Self-efficacy among Adolescents—An Intervention Study." *International Journal of Adolescence and Youth* (2013), doi:10.1080/02673843.2013.779587.

81. Bradley T. Klontz et al. "The Effectiveness of Equine-Assisted Experiential Therapy: Results of an Open Clinical Trial." *Society & Animals* Vol. 15 (2007), pp. 257–67.

82. Canadian Agency for Drugs and Technologies in Health. "Therapy Dogs and Horses for Mental Health: A Review of the Clinical Effectiveness," August 10, 2012. [online]. [cited September 13, 2013]. cadth.ca/media/pdf/htis/aug-2012/RC0381%20Therapy%20Animals%20final.pdf.

83. Erin Russell. "Horses as Healers for Veterans." *Canadian Medical Association Journal* Vol. 185 (2013), p. 1205, doi:10.1503/cmaj.109-4578.

84. Bente Berget et al. "Humans with Mental Disorders Working with Farm Animals." *Occupational Therapy in Mental Health* Vol. 23 (2007), pp. 101–117; Bente Berget and Bjarne O. Braastad. "Animal-assisted Therapy with Farm Animals for Persons with Psychiatric Disorders." *Annali dell'Istituto Superiore di Sanità* Vol. 47 (2011), pp. 384–90; Bente Berget et al. "Animal-assisted Therapy with Farm Animals for Persons with Psychiatric Disorders: Effects on Self-efficacy, Coping Ability and Quality of Life, a Randomized Controlled Trial." *Clinical Practice and Epidemiology in Mental Health* Vol. 4 (2008).

85. Ingeborg Pedersen et al. "Farm Animal-Assisted Intervention for People with Clinical Depression: A Randomized Controlled Trial." *Anthrozoös* Vol. 25 (2012), pp. 149–60.

86. Ingeborg Pedersen et al. "Farm Animal-assisted Intervention: Relationship between Work and Contact with Farm Animals and Change in Depression, Anxiety, and Self-Efficacy Among Persons with Clinical Depression." *Issues in Mental Health Nursing* Vol. 32 (2011), pp. 493–500.

87. Richard Louv. *The Nature Principle: Human Restoration and the End of Nature-deficit Disorder*. Algonquin, 2011, p. 66.

88. Jason Duvall and Rachel Kaplan. *Exploring the Benefits of Outdoor Experiences on Veterans: Report Prepared for the Sierra Club Military Families and Veterans Initiative*, June 2013. [online]. [cited July 25, 2013]. sierraclub.org/military/downloads/Michigan-Final-Research-Report.pdf.

89. Susan Brock and Greg Passey. "The Canadian Military and Veteran Experience," in Scurfield and Platoni, eds. *War Trauma and Its Wake*. See Chapter 4 of *Field Exercises* for the story of CVAF founder Christian McEachern.

90. Ibid., p. 103.

91. Ibid., p. 107.

92. Valvincent Reyes. "Enhancing Resiliency through Creative Outdoor/Adventure and Community-based Programs," in Scurfield and Platoni, eds. *War Trauma and Its Wake*.

93. Keith G. Tidball and Marianne E. Krasny. *Greening in the Red Zone: Disaster, Resilience and Community Greening*. Springer Netherlands, 2014, p. 26.

94. Keith G. Tidball, "Returning Warriors and Environmental Education Opportunities: Outdoor Recreation, Education, and Restoration for Veterans

#CEL002" in Cornell Civic Ecology Lab, ed. *Civic Ecology Lab White Paper Series*. Cornell, 2013. [online]. [cited August 28, 2013]. http://civeco.files .wordpress.com/2013/09/tidball-2013-warriors.pdf.

95. Keith Tidball. Conversation with author, September 4, 2013.

96. Sharon Rogers, David P. Loy and Christina Brown-Bochicchio. "'Sharing a New Foxhole with Friends': The Impact of Outdoor Recreation on Injured Military." unpublished manuscript. [online]. [cited August 25, 2013]. helpkwo.org/files/Sharing%20a%20New%20Foxhole%20with%20 Friends.pdf.

97. Lee Hyer et al. "Effects of Outward Bound Experience as an Adjunct to Inpatient PTSD Treatment of War Veterans." *Journal of Clinical Psychology* Vol. 52 (1996), pp. 263–78.

98. Nevin Harper, Julian Norris and Mark DasTous. "Veterans and the Outward Bound Experience: An Evaluation of Impact and Meaning." *Ecopsychology*, forthcoming. Provided to author via e-mail by Nevin Harper, August 29, 2013.

99. Marc Gelkopf et al. "Nature Adventure Rehabilitation for Combat-related Posttraumatic Chronic Stress Disorder: A Randomized Control Trial." *Psychiatry Research* Vol. 209 (2013), pp. 485–93.

100. Ibid., p. 491.

101. Jacqueline Atkinson. "An Evaluation of the Gardening Leave Project for Ex-military Personnel with PTSD and Other Combat Related Mental Health Problems." Gardening Leave, June 2009. [online]. [cited August 15, 2013]. gardeningleave.org/wp-content/uploads/2009/06/completegl summary.pdf.

102. Sus Sola Corazon et al. "Nature as Therapist: Integrating Permaculture with Mindfulness- and Acceptance-based Therapy in the Danish Healing Forest Garden Nacadia." *European Journal of Psychotherapy & Counselling* Vol. 14 (2012), pp. 335–47.

103. Natalia Pantelidou. "Nacadia, Healing Garden," April 10, 2012. [online]. [cited September 15, 2013]. nataliapantelidou.com/default.aspx?lang=en -GB&page=2&newsid=30#; Dorthe Varning Poulsen. E-mail message to author, September 27, 2013.

104. Billy Briggs. "A different battle: Living with post traumatic stress disorder." *The Scotsman*, June 24, 2012. [online]. [cited October 22, 2013]. scotsman .com/lifestyle/a-different-battle-living-with-post-traumatic-stress-disor der-1-2373409.

105. Anne-Line Ussing. "Pilot Project: Nature Retreat for Veterans." March 2013. Project overview written for the Black Watch Association and provided to author via e-mail by Anne-Line Ussing, October 25, 2013.

Chapter 3

1. All quotations in this chapter are from conversations with Nathan Lewis on November 5, 2012 and August 7, 2013.

Chapter 4

1. All quotations in this chapter are from conversations with Christian McEachern on January 14, 2010 and July 31, 2013 and from e-mails with Christian McEachern on August 4, 2013 and January 11, 2014.
2. Ian Sherrington. This and subsequent quotations from conversation with author, December 15, 2009.
3. Monica Culic. This and subsequent quotations from conversation with author, January 12, 2010.
4. The comments were posted by veteran participants on the CVAF's on-line guest book in 2009 and 2010 at canadianveteranadventurefoundation .com/Guest-Book.html. However, after the CVAF disbanded in 2011, the website is no longer available.
5. Ibid.
6. See Chapter 7 for more about the story of Can Praxis.

Chapter 5

1. All quotations in this chapter are from conversations with Penny Dex on November 16, 2012 and May 8, 2013, and from an e-mail with Penny Dex September 7, 2013.
2. US Department of Labor. "Trauma-Informed Care for Women Veterans Experiencing Homelessness: A Guide for Service Providers." [online]. [cited February 1, 2014]. dol.gov/wb/trauma/traumaguide.htm; James Risen. "Military Has Not Solved Problem of Sexual Assault, Women Say." *New York Times*, November 2, 2012. [online]. [cited February 1, 2014]. nytimes.com/2012/11/02/us/women-in-air-force-say-sexual-misconduct -still-rampant.html.

Chapter 6

1. All quotations in this chapter are from conversations with Deston Denniston on November 20, 2012 and September 4, 2013, and from e-mails with Deston Denniston on December 12, 2012, September 8, 2013, October 17, 2013 and February 1, 2014.
2. More information about the Nisqually Delta Restoration project can be found online at nisquallydeltarestoration.org/ and fws.gov/refuge /Nisqually/.
3. House Committee on Veterans' Affairs. "The Veterans Opportunity to Work Act (The VOW Act) [online]. [cited February 1, 2014]. veterans .house.gov/jobs; US Environmental Protection Agency. "AG 101: De-

mographics." [online]. [cited February 1, 2014]. epa.gov/oecaagct/ag101
/demographics.html; Bloomberg News. "Number of U.S. Farms Fell
to Six-Year Low in 2012, USDA Says." [online]. [cited February 1, 2014].
bloomberg.com/news/2013-02-19/number-of-u-s-farms-fell-to-six-year
-low-in-2012-usda-says-1-.html.

4. Abundance Permaculture. "Seedballs."[online]. [cited September 7, 2013].
abundancepermaculture.com/seedballs.

Chapter 7

1. All quotations in this chapter are from conversations with Steve Critchley
on June 25, 2013, and Jim Marland on June 26, 2013, and from e-mails with
Steve Critchley on July 30, 2013 and August 14, 2013, and from an e-mail
with Jim Marland on August 10, 2013.

2. Equine-Assisted Learning is a Canadian federal government approved and
recognized program.

3. Canada's national breed: see canadianhorsebreeders.com and lechevalcan
adien.ca/indexen.htm.

4. Steven Blaney was Canada's Minister of Veterans Affairs from May 18, 2011
to July 14, 2013.

5. Scott Maxwell. Conversation with author, June 27, 2013.

Chapter 8

1. All quotations in this chapter are from conversations with Christopher
Brown on November 23, 2012 and July 11, 2013, and from an e-mail with
Christopher Brown on August 3, 2013.

2. Chris has written several blog entries about his experiences. See Chris
Brown. "A Burden We Share." [online]. [cited February 4, 2014]. growing
veterans.org/a-burden-we-share; Chris Brown. "'Still There'—The Song
That Sustains." [online]. [cited February 4, 2014]. growingveterans.org
/stillthere.

3. Growing Veterans. "Our Mission." [online]. [cited February 4, 2014].
growingveterans.org/overview/.

4. Growing Veterans. "The Horn." [online]. [cited February 4, 2014]. growing
veterans.org/the-horn/.

5. Growing Veterans. "Op Wire." [online]. [cited February 4, 2014]. growing
veterans.org/opwire/.

Chapter 9

1. All quotations in this chapter are from conversations with Gordon
Cousins on January 27, 2010, October 18, 2011 and September 5, 2013, and
from e-mails with Gordon Cousins on June 6, 2011 and November 21,
2011.

Chapter 10

1. Shepherd Bliss has written a number of articles about his experiences. All quotations in this chapter not otherwise referenced are from conversations with Shepherd Bliss on July 28, 2011 and July 11, 2013, and from an e-mail with Shepherd Bliss on August 19, 2013.

2. Shepherd Bliss. "The Veterans Writing Group and the Military Community." *Communities Magazine* #159 (Summer 2013). [online]. [cited July 25, 2013]. communities.ic.org/articles/1673/The_Veterans_Writing_Group _and_the_Military_Community.

3. See Chapter 1 for a description of the various and changing terminologies used to describe stress injuries.

4. Shepherd Bliss. "Sound Shy" in Kingston, ed. Veterans of War, Veterans of Peace, p. 23. vowvop.org.

5. Ibid.

6. Ibid., p. 24.

7. Ibid., p. 25.

8. Shepherd Bliss. "In Praise of Sweet Darkness." in Buzzell and Chalquist, eds. *Ecotherapy*, p. 174.

9. Shepherd Bliss. "Learning from the Community of the Land." Smirking Chimp website, June 19, 2011. [online]. [cited June 20, 2013]. smirking chimp.com/thread/shepherd-bliss/36852/learning-from-the-community -of-the-land.

10. "In our group," Shepherd told me, "we don't judge people. They tell their story. We let them tell their story. And then sometimes we write somebody's story because they can't."

11. Bliss, "In Praise of Sweet Darkness," p. 178.

12. Ibid. p. 177.

13. Bliss, "Learning from the Community of the Land."

14. Bliss, "In Praise of Sweet Darkness," p. 175.

15. Shepherd Bliss. "Farms Heal—Agrotherapy." CounterCurrents.org, February 2, 2009. [online]. [cited June 20, 2013]. countercurrents.org/bliss020 209.htm.

16. Ibid.

17. See Chapter 11 for more information about green care.

Chapter 11

1. Terry Hartig and Clare Cooper Marcus. "Healing Gardens—Places for Nature in Health Care." *The Lancet, Medicine and Creativity* 368 (2006), p. s37.

2. Rachel Hine, Jo Peacock and Jules Pretty. "Care Farming in the UK: Contexts, Benefits and Links with Therapeutic Communities." *Therapeutic Communities* Vol. 29 (2008), pp. 245–60; Mind, *Ecotherapy*.

3. Dorit Karla Haubenhofer et al. "The Development of Green Care in Western European Countries." *EXPLORE: The Journal of Science and Healing* Vol. 6 (2010), pp. 106–11.

4. Mind, *Ecotherapy*, p. 7.

5. The paper used to print this book is 100% post-consumer, recycled, FSC-certified.

6. Joe Sempik, Rachel Hine and Deborah Wilcox, eds. *Green Care: A Conceptual Framework. A Report of the Working Group on the Health Benefits of Green Care, COST Action 866, Green Care in Agriculture.* Centre for Child and Family Research, Loughborough University, 2010. [online]. [cited September 10, 2013]. umb.no/statisk/greencare/green_carea_conceptual_framework.pdf.

7. Joost Dessein and Bettina B. Bock, eds. *The Economics of Green Care in Agriculture.* COST Action 866, Green Care in Agriculture. Loughborough University, 2010, p. 11.

8. European Cooperation in Science and Technology. *Green Care in Agriculture.* [online]. [cited September 10, 2013]. cost.eu/domains_actions/fa/Actions/866.

9. Marjolein Elings and Jan Hassink. "Green Care Farms, a Safe Community between Illness or Addiction and the Wider Society." *Therapeutic Communities* Vol. 29 (2008), pp. 310–22.

10. Francesco Di Iacovo and Deirdre O'Connor, eds. *Supporting Policies for Social Farming in Europe: Progressing Multifunctionality in Responsive Rural Areas.* Press Service srl, Sesto Fiorentino (FI), 2009, p. 120. [online]. [cited August 16, 2011]. sofar.unipi.it/index_file/arsia_So.Far-EU_def.pdf.

11. Mind, *Ecotherapy*.

12. Bettina B. Bock and Simon J. Oosting. "A Classification of Green Care Arrangements in Europe" in Dessein and Bock, eds. *The Economics of Green Care in Agriculture.*

13. Ibid., p. 19.

14. Evy Mettepenningen et al. "Green Care in the Framework of Multifunctional Agriculture" in Dessein and Bock, eds. *The Economics of Green Care in Agriculture*, p. 47.

15. Ibid., p. 52.

16. Dessein and Bock, eds., *The Economics of Green Care in Agriculture.*

17. Joost Dessein, Bettina B. Bock and Michiel P. M. M. de Kroma. "Investigating the Limits of Multifunctional Agriculture as the Dominant Frame for Green Care in Agriculture in Flanders and the Netherlands." *Journal of Rural Studies* Vol. 32 (2013), pp. 50–59.

18. Bock and Oosting, "A Classification of Green Care Arrangements."

19. Di Iacovo and O'Connor, eds., *Supporting Policies for Social Farming in Europe.*

20. Berlin Center for Torture Victims. "Healing Garden." [online]. [cited September 2, 2011]. bzfo.de/work/services/garden.html.

21. Haubenhofer et al., "The Development of Green Care."

22. Bock and Oosting, "A Classification of Green Care Arrangements."

23. Rachel Hine, Jo Peacock and Jules Pretty. *Care Farming in the UK: Evidence and Opportunities.* Report for the National Care Farming Initiative (UK), 2008. [online]. [cited September 10, 2013]. carefarmingadvocacy.org/Care farmingintheUKFINALJan08.pdf.

24. Haubenhofer et al., "The Development of Green Care."

25. Di Iacovo and O'Connor, eds., *Supporting Policies for Social Farming in Europe.*

26. Bock and Oosting, "A Classification of Green Care Arrangements," p. 22.

27. Tidball, conversation with author.

28. Shirley Fox. "Welcoming Heroes Home with a Very Special Garden." Returning Heroes Home, August 19, 2013. [online]. [cited September 13, 2013]. returningheroeshome.org/archive/2013/08/19/welcoming-heroes-home-very-special-garden; Therapeutic Landscapes Network. "The Warrior and Family Support Center—A Green Haven in San Antonio, TX." [online]. [cited September 13, 2013]. healinglandscapes.org/blog/2012/11/the-warrior-and-family-support-center-a-green-haven-in-san-antonio-tx.

29. Richard J. Onken. "A Rigorous Approach to Evidence-Based Design." *Healthcare Design,* January 3, 2012. [online]. [cited September 13, 2013]. healthcaredesignmagazine.com/article/rigorous-approach-evidence-based-design?page=2.

30. David P. Ball. "Cops Go beyond the Kale of Duty." *24 Hours Vancouver,* August 21, 2013. [online]. [cited August 30, 2013]. vancouver.24hrs.ca/2013/08/21/cops-go-beyond-the-kale-of-duty.

31. Sarah Wash. "The Healing Power of Flowers: Torture Victims Turn to Gardens for Hope." *Utne Reader* (March/April 2006). [online]. [cited September 2, 2011]. utne.com/community/thehealingpoweroflowers.aspx.

32. Ibid.

33. Mitchell Hewson. "Horticultural Therapy and Post Traumatic Stress Recovery." *Journal of Therapeutic Horticulture* Vol. XII (2001), pp. 44–47; Homewood Health Centre. "Program for Traumatic Stress Recovery." [online]. [cited September 14, 2013]. homewood.org/programs-and-services/post-traumatic-stress-recovery.

34. Linford, *Warrior Rising,* p. 350.

35. Chris Linford. Conversation with author, July 25, 2013.

36. Farmer Veteran Coalition. [online]. [cited February 8, 2014]. farmvetco.org.

37. Christopher, conversation with author.

38. Ibid.

39. Sarah Elton. *Consumed: Food for a Finite Planet.* HarperCollins, 2013, p. 92.

40. Nadia El-Hage Scialabba. "Organic Agriculture and Food Security." Paper presented at the International Conference on Organic Agriculture and Food Security, May 5–7, 2007, p. 13. [online]. [cited October 16, 2013]. ftp.fao.org/paia/organicag/ofs/OFS-2007-5.pdf.

41. Nebraska College of Technical Agriculture. "Combat Boots to Cowboy Boots." [online]. [cited February 8, 2014]. ncta.unl.edu/combatcowboy boots.

42. Archi's Acres. "VSAT Program." [online]. [cited September 28, 2013]. archisacres.com/page/vsat-program.

43. Patricia Leigh Brown. "Helping Soldiers Trade Their Swords for Plows." *New York Times*, February 5, 2011. [online]. [cited July 20, 2011]. nytimes .com/2011/02/06/us/06vets.html.

44. Ibid.

45. Farmer Veteran Coalition. "Farming Project Invites Veterans to Work and Learn." Press Release, April 23, 2010. [online]. [cited September 28, 2013]. prlog.org/10644284 farming-project-invites-veterans-to-work-and-learn .html.

46. Veterans Farm. *WVFV Veterans Farm.* Video, August 1, 2010. [online]. [cited September 28, 2013]. youtube.com/watch?v=9Rr1WpOVMIc.

47. Barbara Seymour, producer. *Vets' Garden, Westwood.* Video, 2009. [online]. [cited January 3, 2012]. youtube.com/watch?v=eir1hzvAX-o&feature =related.

48. Maria Papadopoulos. *Healing Greens: Local Vets Find Solace in Horticultural Therapy.* Video, *The Enterprise of Brockton, Massachusetts,* August 31, 2008. [online]. [cited January 3, 2012]. youtube.com/watch?v=1jkoU-_Gpko& NR=1.

49. Erving Goffman. *Asylums: Essays on the Social Situation of Mental Patients and Other Inmates.* Aldine, 1962.

50. Joshua S. Goldstein. *War and Gender: How Gender Shapes the War System and Vice Versa.* Cambridge, 2001.

51. Renate Cervinka, Kathrin Röderer and Elisabeth Hefler. "Are Nature Lovers Happy? On Various Indicators of Well-being and Connectedness with Nature." *Journal of Health Psychology* Vol. 17 (2012), pp. 379–88.

52. Mary Cole and Maureen Howard. "Animal-Assisted Therapy: Benefits and Challenges" in Martin Grassberger et al., eds. *Biotherapy—History, Principles and Practice: A Practical Guide to the Diagnosis and Treatment of Disease using Living Organisms.* Springer, 2013.

53. Herman, *Trauma and Recovery.*

54. Sternberg, *Healing Spaces,* p. 230.

55. Lambert, conversation with author.

56. Lambert, *Lifting Depression.*

57. Lambert, conversation with author.

58. Christopher, conversation with author.

59. Lambert, conversation with author.

60. Fisher, *Radical Ecopsychology*, p. 109.

61. Helphand, *Defiant Gardens*, pp. 230–31.

62. Kurt Hoelting. *The Circumference of Home: One Man's Yearlong Quest for a Radically Local Life*. Da Capo, 2010.

63. Inside Passages website. [online]. [cited September 20, 2013]. inside passages.com.

64. Kurt Hoelting, conversation with author, September 29, 2011. Kurt edited the section about him included in this chapter, and the author received those revisions September 25, 2013 and September 28, 2013.

65. VA Puget Sound Health Care System. "Mindfulness Based Stress Reduction." [online]. [cited September 20, 2013]. pugetsound.va.gov/services /mindfulness.asp.

66. Center for Mindfulness in Medicine, Health Care, and Society website. [online]. [cited September 20, 2013]. umassmed.edu/content.aspx?id =41252.

67. Hoelting, conversation with author.

68. Ibid.

69. Ibid.

70. Tidball, conversation with author.

71. Joe Sempik. "Green Care: A Natural Resource for Therapeutic Communities?" *Therapeutic Communities* Vol. 29 (2008), p. 225.

72. Helphand, *Defiant Gardens*, p. 212.

APPENDIX 1:
RESOURCES FOR VETERANS

As outlined in Chapter 11, there is no standard for green care in North America. On the one hand, this means that veterans with a vision can create peer-support programs for other veterans without a lot of bureaucracy and paperwork. On the other hand, it makes it difficult to investigate, evaluate and advocate for specific programs and groups.

The resources in this Appendix represent a sample of possible starting places for you and/or your loved ones. It includes contact information for a variety of veterans' programs in both the US and Canada (current as of Fall 2013). It also includes general information for those new to gardening.

Please check into the programs further to determine whether they are a good fit for you. You may wish to consult with a physician or other health care provider about the appropriateness of any program, service or activity.

The Field Exercises website (fieldexercises.com) contains an up-to-date and more comprehensive list of veterans' programs, as well as links to gardening information and news articles about veterans' involvement in green care activities.

UNITED STATES
Programs for Veterans
Farmer Veteran Coalition
The Farmer Veteran Coalition (FVC) is a not-for-profit organization that connects military veterans with opportunities for employment, training and places to heal on farms in the US. FVC works with veterans in 48 states to provide farming education and veteran assistance.
web: farmvetco.org

Veterans Farm
The Veterans Farm, based in Jacksonville, Florida, helps disabled combat veterans reintegrate into society through horticulture therapy. In conjunction with The Mission Continues, the Veterans Farm provides a six-month fellowship program to promote and support agro-entrepreneurship and ecological horticulture.

e-mail: info@veteransfarm.com
web: veteransfarm.org

Archi's Acres

Archi's Acres, based in Escondido, California, offers the Veterans Sustainable Agriculture Training (VSAT) program, an intensive six-week agriculture entrepreneur program. The program has more than 200 graduates, and assists in job placement and business creation after classes end. The cost is US$4500.00 (partial tuition assistance may be available on a case-by-case basis).
web: archisacres.com

Growing Veterans

Growing Veterans, based in Bellingham, Washington, works to harness the skills, energy and passion of military veterans to support and strengthen the sustainable agriculture movement. The non-profit organization operates a small farm, which hosts veterans as volunteers, interns and fellows.
e-mail: staff@growingveterans.org
web: growingveterans.org

Veterans' Sanctuary

The non-profit Veterans' Sanctuary, based in Ithaca, New York, offers a peer-based, holistic program that supports veterans as they transition from combat to civilian life. The three-fold program includes a community garden, combat paper making and a bimonthly veterans' writing group.
e-mail: Veterans.Sanctuary@gmail.com
web: veteranssanctuary.blogspot.com

Boots to Roots (Doug Fir Veterans)

Based in Portland, Oregon, Boots to Roots is Doug Fir Veterans' pilot transition program, which works to provide veterans with permaculture-based education, employment and therapy opportunities.
web: dougfirveterans.com

Outward Bound for Veterans

Outward Bound for Veterans supports returning service members and recent veterans in readjusting to life at home through fully funded wilderness courses that draw on the healing benefit of teamwork and challenge in the natural world.
e-mail: cspangler@outwardbound.org
web: outwardbound.org/veteran-adventures/outward-bound-for-veterans

Sierra Club Military Outdoors

Sierra Club Military Outdoors provides a variety of opportunities for military

service members and their families to find adventure, camaraderie, a sense of mission and relaxation through outdoor experiences.
e-mail: stacy.bare@sierraclub.org; or joshua.brandon@sierraclub.org
web: sierraclub.org/military

Disabled Veterans SCUBA Project
The Disabled Veterans SCUBA Project serves disabled veterans by helping them experience the camaraderie of SCUBA diving and the underwater world.
e-mail: president@dvsp.us
web: dvsp.us

The Pathway Home
The Pathway Home offers a residential program involving multiple holistic methods to help those impacted by post-combat mental health challenges to successfully return to civilian life. The program is supported by private grants, donations and fundraising. Residents have the opportunity to be matched with a service dog.
e-mail: fred.gusman@thepathwayhome.org
web: thepathwayhome.org

National Military Family Association—Operation Purple Program
Operation Purple Family Retreats
Operation Purple Family Retreats provide military families with the opportunity to reconnect as a family. Family retreats use a "camp" approach to bring families to outdoor locations where they enjoy family-oriented activities, make new shared memories and spend quality time together.
e-mail: OPC@MilitaryFamily.org
web: militaryfamily.org/our-programs/operation-purple/family-retreats

Operation Purple Camp
Operation Purple Camp brings together military children from all ranks and services for a summer camp experience in locations throughout the US.
e-mail: OPC@MilitaryFamily.org
web: militaryfamily.org/our-programs/operation-purple/traditional-camps

Operation Purple Healing Adventures
Operation Purple Healing Adventures is a retreat program that supports wounded service members and their families. It combines family-focused activities with outdoor exploration to encourage each family's growth; activities include climbing, hiking, canoeing and more.
e-mail: OPC@MilitaryFamily.org
web: militaryfamily.org/our-programs/operation-purple/wounded-warriors
-families

Wounded Warrior Project—Project Odyssey
Project Odyssey supports veterans in overcoming combat stress through outdoor rehabilitative retreats in various regions in the US. Activities encourage connection with nature, peers, staff and trained counselors.
e-mail: projectodyssey@woundedwarriorproject.org.
web: woundedwarriorproject.org/programs/combat-stress-recovery-program/project-odyssey.aspx

Higher Ground Military Programs
Higher Ground (HG) hosts eight week-long sports camps annually, free of charge, to veterans and their supporters. Camps serve 8–10 participants and are designed for specific populations (couples, men, women); activities include snow sports, rafting, water sports and fly fishing.
e-mail: info@HigherGroundSV.com
web: highergroundsv.org/military_programs

Project Sanctuary
Project Sanctuary, based in Colorado, provides therapeutic retreats throughout the year. These enable members of military families to reconnect through shared activities and educational programs. Families are further supported by a two-year follow-up program.
e-mail: Info@ProjectSanctuary.us
web: projectsanctuary.us

Veterans Expeditions
Veterans Expeditions is a Colorado-based, veteran-run non-profit that uses wilderness challenges to connect veterans, create community and raise awareness.
e-mail: nick@vetexpeditions.com
web: vetexpeditions.com

Warrior Hike
Warrior Hike has partnered with the Appalachian Trail Conservancy, the Continental Divide Trail Coalition and the Pacific Crest Trail Association to create the "Walk Off the War" Program. The program offers combat veterans transitioning from their military service an opportunity to thru-hike national scenic trails in the US.
e-mail: warriorhike@gmail.com
web: warriorhike.com

Project Healing Waters Fly Fishing Inc.
Project Healing Waters Fly Fishing is dedicated to rehabilitation through fly fishing education and outings. Services and programs are offered free of charge to injured military service personnel and disabled veterans throughout the US.

e-mail: admin@projecthealingwaters.org
web: projecthealingwaters.org

Saratoga WarHorse

Saratoga WarHorse, based in Saratoga Springs, New York, assists veterans and victims of trauma suffering from psychological wounds through providing a confidential, action-based, equine-based experience. Saratoga WarHorse covers the costs of transportation, lodging, food and tuition for all veterans attending its programs.
e-mail: bob@saratogawarhorse.com
web: saratogawarhorse.com

Saddles for Soldiers

Saddles for Soldiers is operated by the Shadow Hills Riding Club, a PATH International Premier Accredited Center in Shadow Hills, California. Through interacting with horses, US veterans and their families work toward reestablishing life skills and adjusting to civilian life after return from combat.
email: info@saddlesforsoldiers.org
web: saddlesforsoldiers.org

Horses for Heroes—New Mexico, Inc.

Horses For Heroes—New Mexico offers Cowboy Up!, a unique horsemanship, wellness and skill set restructuring program based in Santa Fe. The Cowboy Up! program is free to both male and female OIF, OEF and OND veterans as well as active military who have sustained physical injuries or combat trauma during their service.
e-mail: info@horsesforheroes.org
web: horsesforheroes.org

Horses Building Communities

Horses Building Communities serves Sonoma County, California, and outlying areas. Its therapeutic equine program is designed to help military personnel and their families improve interpersonal relationships and reconnect with their communities, from pre-deployment through homecoming.
e-mail: dp@horsesbuildingcommunities.org
web: horsesbuildingcommunities.org

Combat Boots to Cowboy Boots

Combat Boots to Cowboy Boots is a University of Nebraska—Nebraska College of Technical Agriculture (NCTA) program designed to assist eligible military personnel, their families and armed forces veterans to find next careers as farmers, ranchers or business entrepreneurs.
web: ncta.unl.edu/combatcowboyboots

Veterans Conservation Corps of Chicagoland
The VCC's mission is to make a positive difference both in the lives of veterans and in the landscapes in which they live. VCC members accomplish this through hands-on restoration of degraded natural lands.
e-mail: haberthurben@kaneforest.com
Facebook: facebook.com/VeteransConservationCorps

Wounded Warriors in Action Foundation, Inc.
The Wounded Warriors in Action Foundation Inc. (WWIA), based in Apollo Beach, Florida, serves combat-wounded Purple Heart recipients. Hunting and fishing programs encourage independence and connection with community while promoting healing and wellness through camaraderie and a shared passion for the outdoors.
e-mail: info@wwiaf.org
web: wwiaf.org

Keeping Warriors Outdoors
Each year, Keeping Warriors Outdoors (KWO), based in Virginia, enables 20 wounded warriors to take an initial week-long hiatus from hospital life for an all-expenses-paid outdoor adventure. KWO provides formal instruction on archery, hunting, fishing and other outdoor activities before participants put their new skills to work in tournaments. All gear is provided. Veterans then continue to participate in KWO-sponsored hunting and fishing expeditions throughout the year.
web: helpkwo.org

CANADA

Wounded Warriors Canada
Wounded Warriors Canada is a non-profit organization that helps Canadian Forces members (full-time and reservists) who have been wounded or injured in their service to Canada. Wounded Warriors Canada funds a variety of programs, including Courageous Companions Elite K-9 Service Dogs and Can Praxis (see below). They also sponsor the annual Wounded Warriors Weekend.
e-mail: info@woundedwarriors.ca
web: woundedwarriors.ca

Courageous Companions Elite K-9 Service Dogs
Courageous Companions is a world leader in service dog training and education. The group trains dogs to work specifically with veterans suffering from post-traumatic stress disorder.
email: GL@msar.ca
web: msar.ca

Can Praxis

The Can Praxis equine therapy program relies on the natural instincts of horses and staff expertise in communication, conflict resolution and team-building to support veterans in regaining family relationships, as well as to promote personal renewal and improved quality of life. All programs are offered free of charge to Canadian Forces veterans.

email: steve@canpraxis.com, or admin@canpraxis.com

Facebook: facebook.com/CanPraxis

Citadel Canine Society

Citadel Canine Society is a CRA-registered non-profit society that trains, tests and provides service or companion dogs at no charge to new veterans, police officers and other first responders dealing with PTSD. Citadel Canine often uses rescue dogs saved from animal shelters.

e-mail: info@citadelcanine.com

web: citadelcanine.com

Outward Bound Canada—Veterans' Programs

Outward Bound Canada offers one week, adventure-based resiliency training for Canadian Forces veterans in the Canadian Rockies. These programs are open to all current and former Canadian Forces members; programs provide an opportunity to connect with other veterans in a supportive environment. Course tuition and travel costs are covered; there is no cost to participate on this program.

email: veterans@outwardbound.ca

web: outwardbound.ca

Project Healing Waters Fly Fishing Canada

Project Healing Waters Fly Fishing Canada is dedicated to the physical and emotional rehabilitation of disabled military personnel and veterans through fly fishing and fly-tying education and outings. With locations throughout Canada, the program is available at no cost to beginners as well as to experienced fly fishers wanting to adapt their skills to their new abilities.

web: projecthealingwaters.ca

APPENDIX 2:
GARDENING ON YOUR OWN
OR WITH YOUR FAMILY

Some of the veterans featured in *Field Exercises* started their journeys toward healing through gardening. Growing flowers and trees can contribute aesthetically to your surroundings and contribute a wide ecological function by providing home and food for birds, bees, insects and animals. Many veterans find growing food to be important because it allows them to nourish their own bodies and also to nourish other people, including their family, friends and allies in their communities.

Growing food is something that you can do easily and cheaply, on your own or with others. Once established, you might even begin to learn how to save your own seeds and branch out into other areas, such as permaculture. You can grow food at a very small scale or expand your efforts as you gain more confidence and knowledge about what is required. (Visit fieldexercises.com for links and websites that might be helpful to beginning gardeners.)

It is possible to grow plants and food in a variety of locations, including inside your apartment or house, on your balcony, in your backyard (or front yard, although some communities have bylaws that prevent front yard vegetable gardening), in a community garden plot, through horticultural therapy programs and even by connecting with farms in your area. If you live in the US, veteran-owned farms are emerging all over the country, and many welcome volunteers.

If you are new to gardening and intend to try it on your own, you might consider calling or visiting your local garden center for advice, finding gardening books and/or magazines written specifically for your region or doing some Internet research. If you are new to growing food, it takes some practice. Here are some things you'll need to consider:

What Is Your Gardening Zone?
The length of the growing season and the types of plants that grow well varies by gardening zone. In particular, you'll want to know how many days in your region are frost-free per year, on average. Some plants grow better in cooler weather

while others do best when it's hot. Lettuce, radishes, beans and carrots tend to grow easily during the summer months in most climates.

How Much Space Do You Have?

Some plants (such as carrots, potatoes, beets) require substantial root space or extensive above-ground growing space (such as pumpkins, zucchinis).

What Time of Year Is It?

If you live in the northern US or Canada and are reading this book in November, it's not a good time to start growing fruits and vegetables. That said, many gardeners do start seeds indoors, either in a window or beneath grow lights. This helps to extend the growing season, since when the time comes, you can plant out mature seedlings. Most nurseries sell starter trays to be used for this purpose, but you can also create your own out of newspapers, egg cartons or even egg shells.

How Much Sun Will Your Plants Get?

All plants require sun, but some do better than others in shadier areas. If you have a spot that receives only a few hours of sun per day, it's best not to plant crops that produce fruit (such as tomatoes, eggplant and peppers). Leafy vegetables, such as kale, arugula, spinach and lettuce, as well as root vegetables, such as carrots and beets, are more able to tolerate shade. Just be aware that it might take longer for your crop to mature in lower light conditions.

What If You Don't Have Access
to an Outdoor Space for Growing?

If you don't have access to an outdoor space, there are indoor experiments you might try, such as regrowing food from kitchen scraps. For example, the next time you have celery, cut the stalks from their base, and instead of discarding the base, place it cut ends up in a shallow dish of water—just enough water to cover the base, but not the top—in a window or area with bright sunlight. Replace the water every day or two (do not let it dry out). After a few days, you'll notice that the old cut stalks have started to whither, but there will be new growth at the center of the stalk. Once the new growth is an inch high, you can plant the whole base in a pot with soil (cover everything except the new leaves) and water regularly. Eventually, you will be able to harvest stalks as you need them. Other vegetables can be regrown in a similar way, including pineapple, ginger, romaine lettuce, leeks and green onions. You can also grow plants such as avocados and even lemons and oranges from their seeds.

Indoor vegetable gardening is also growing in popularity. Some vegetables can be grown easily in a window sill, including leafy greens such as lettuce and spinach, and fast-growing varieties of radishes that don't require much root space. If you don't want to invest in pots, you can even repurpose items from your kitchen, such as clean empty milk cartons since these plants don't have extensive root systems. Just be sure to punch drainage holes in the bottom, allowing the impromptu pots to drain onto a plate or pan. If you are feeling adventurous, you might also experiment with carrots, beets, tomatoes, potatoes, beans and peppers in containers. These plants have more extensive root systems and require larger pots. They also have more extensive light requirements.

Most importantly:

- **Start small:** Many of us have a tendency to leap into something like this full steam ahead, but most veterans I talked with recommended starting with small and manageable projects.
- **Don't get discouraged:** Many gardeners can attest to the importance of trial and error. If at first you don't succeed, do some research into what went wrong. Check with your local garden center, gardening books or gardening websites.
- **Choose something that fits your abilities:** You can still garden with physical injuries. If you are in a wheelchair, for example, a garden bed on the ground likely won't work for you; however, with the support of family and friends, there are plenty of freely available designs on the Internet for building raised garden beds compatible with wheelchairs, as well as gardening tables and vertical wall gardens. If you prefer not to rely on external help, you might try using containers and hanging planters—just make sure they are wide enough and hold enough dirt so that they don't dry out too quickly. There are also gardening tools designed specifically for people with physical disabilities.

INDEX

If you have enjoyed *Field Exercises*,
you might also enjoy other

Books to Build a New Society

Our books provide positive solutions for people who want to
make a difference. We specialize in:

**Sustainable Living • Green Building • Peak Oil •
Renewable Energy • Environment & Economy Natural
Building & Appropriate Technology Progressive Leadership
• Resistance and Community Educational & Parenting Resources**

New Society Publishers

ENVIRONMENTAL BENEFITS STATEMENT

New Society Publishers has chosen to produce this book on recycled
paper made with **100% post consumer waste**, processed chlorine
free, and old growth free.

For every 5,000 books printed, New Society saves the following
resources:[1]

25	Trees
2,264	Pounds of Solid Waste
2,491	Gallons of Water
3,249	Kilowatt Hours of Electricity
4,115	Pounds of Greenhouse Gases
18	Pounds of HAPs, VOCs, and AOX Combined
6	Cubic Yards of Landfill Space

[1]Environmental benefits are calculated based on research done by the
Environmental Defense Fund and other members of the Paper Task Force who study
the environmental impacts of the paper industry

For a full list of NSP's titles, please call 1-800-567-6772 *or check out our website* at:

www.newsociety.com

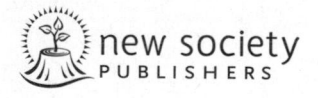

new society
PUBLISHERS

If you have enjoyed *Field Exercises*,
you might also enjoy other

BOOKS TO BUILD A NEW SOCIETY

Our books provide positive solutions for people who want to
make a difference. We specialize in:

**Sustainable Living • Green Building • Peak Oil •
Renewable Energy • Environment & Economy Natural
Building & Appropriate Technology Progressive Leadership
• Resistance and Community Educational & Parenting Resources**

New Society Publishers

ENVIRONMENTAL BENEFITS STATEMENT

New Society Publishers has chosen to produce this book on recycled
paper made with **100% post consumer waste**, processed chlorine
free, and old growth free.

For every 5,000 books printed, New Society saves the following
resources:[1]

25	Trees
2,264	Pounds of Solid Waste
2,491	Gallons of Water
3,249	Kilowatt Hours of Electricity
4,115	Pounds of Greenhouse Gases
18	Pounds of HAPs, VOCs, and AOX Combined
6	Cubic Yards of Landfill Space

[1]Environmental benefits are calculated based on research done by the
Environmental Defense Fund and other members of the Paper Task Force who study
the environmental impacts of the paper industry.

For a full list of NSP's titles, please call 1-800-567-6772 *or check out our website* at:

www.newsociety.com

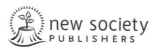

new society
PUBLISHERS

ABOUT THE AUTHOR

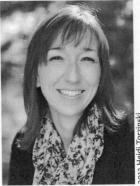

STEPHANIE WESTLUND holds a PhD in Peace and Conflict Studies, and was the 2012-2013 Global Citizenship Research Fellow in the Consortium for Peace Studies at the University of Calgary. She has been conducting research with veterans since 2009, and continues to be inspired by their courage and personal resolve to move through pain toward recovery, and their unrelenting desire to serve their communities. Stephanie blogs about the human-nature relationship at Our Common Nature www.ourcommonnature.blogspot.com